The Ultimate Guide to Pregnancy for Lesbians

The Ultimate Guide to Pregnancy for Lesbians

How to Stay Sane and Care for Yourself
from Preconception Through Birth

SECOND EDITION

by Rachel Pepper

CLEIS
PRESS

Published in the United States by Cleis Press Inc.,
P.O. Box 14697, San Francisco, California 94114.

Printed in the United States.
Cover design: Scott Idleman
Cover photo: Getty Images
Author photo: Debra St. John
Book design: Karen Quigg
Cleis Press logo art: Juana Alicia
10 9 8 7 6 5 4 3 2 1

Library of Congress Cataloging-in-Publication Data

Pepper, Rachel.
    The ultimate guide to pregnancy for lesbians : how to stay sane and care for yourself from preconception through birth / by Rachel Pepper.— 2nd ed.
        p. cm.
    Includes bibliographical references and index.
    ISBN 1-57344-216-X (pbk. : alk. paper)
    1. Pregnancy—Miscellanea. 2. Lesbian mothers—Health and hygiene—Miscellanea.
I. Title.
    RG556P47 2005
    618.2—dc22   2005020750

*I dedicate this book, again, to every lesbian dreaming baby dreams.
This second edition is also dedicated to the many dyke daddies and tranny pops
out there, arms and hearts so wide open. This book is for all of you, with love.
And as before, it's especially for my own daughter, Frances Ariel,
who finally made my own baby dreams come true.*

ACKNOWLEDGMENTS

For help in updating this edition, I would like to thank Cathy Winks and the Sperm Bank of California; Aimee Gelnaw of the Family Pride Coalition; Kate Kendell, Director of the National Center for Lesbian Rights; midwife Deborah Simone; and all the moms who sent me comments and quotes for use in this edition.

Big thanks to Linda L. Anderson and Jolisa Gracewood for reading the manuscript and making so many thoughtful suggestions. I really, really owe you gals.

My daughter, Frances, deserves kudos here for dealing with a mom always yelling, "Don't bug me, I'm writing!" This little angel did hundreds of art projects and watched lots of movies and PBS so I could finish this edition. It's not always easy being the kid of a single mom, especially one on deadline. Thanks, babe.

Contents

Why a Second Edition?

You hold in your hands the second edition of the world's first-ever pregnancy book for lesbians. The first edition, released in 1999, was inspired by a series of articles I wrote in *Curve* magazine in 1998 about my attempts at conception. Back then, when I was going through the many issues discussed in this book's pages, there was no lesbian pregnancy book to read, and I felt very alone in my journey. True, there were, and still are, good books for lesbians considering parenthood, as well as for lesbians who are already raising children. The lack of information for the specific journey a lesbian will find herself on during her path to pregnancy resulted in the first edition of my book, which was read by thousands of women.

Perhaps as a direct result of my book and others that followed, much has changed in the lesbian nation. More and more lesbians are considering parenthood and feeling supported in their decision to have children. Where even a few years ago a woman might be the pioneer in her peer group if she considered parenthood, now it is the norm in certain circles. Children are everywhere in the lesbian community. They run rampant in sacred lesbian enclaves like the Michigan Womyn's Music Festival, they are at Pride celebrations and film festivals, and childcare centers and groups for parents are provided at many gay and lesbian centers and events across the country. Our children are our prized and valued community members—for some of us, the heart and soul of the queer community. And where once, in darker days, AIDS was the common ground that brought gay men and lesbians together, now parenting and the love of our children is one happy thread that ties together our community.

So, if my book has been so successful, why revise it? First, a lot can change in six years. I wrote most of the first edition while I was still pregnant, and finished it when my daughter, Frances, was merely months old. My daughter is now almost seven—practically a full-fledged tween. I like to feel that she and I have raised each other well, and this book will benefit from the added wisdom she has brought to my life.

Second, the legal status of lesbian parents continues to shift. This edition addresses our legal concerns with the most current information available, courtesy of Kate Kendell of the National Center for Lesbian Rights (NCLR).

Third, readers of the second edition are far more Internet savvy than ever before. This edition includes lots of new online resources, including websites, bulletin boards, and blogs. Even sperm banks are now online, with sites that list their donors' availability based on hourly supply checks.

This second edition of *The Ultimate Guide to Pregnancy for Lesbians* is revised from front cover to back, with lots of new information on almost every page. You will find a greatly expanded chapter on how to decide if you're ready for parenthood, lots more info on sperm banks and choosing a donor, revised sections on every trimester of pregnancy, clearer explanations of the birth experience, and extra support for surviving your newborn, all from someone who's been there.

The resources section has also been completely revamped, filling out the book like a well-rounded, pregnant lesbian belly.

I hope you enjoy reading my book, and that it helps you on your path to parenthood. As always, and with an eye to future generations of this book, I look forward to hearing from you. Feel free to send me comments or suggestions for future editions, pictures of your beautiful babies, or simply share your own journey toward and into motherhood at bernalbks@aol.com.

Best wishes,
Rachel Pepper
July, 2005

Chapter

1

So You Wanna Be a Mama

Welcome to the wacky world of lesbian conception and pregnancy! I suspect, given my own experience, that you have only a vague notion at this point of what you're getting yourself into. Getting pregnant is usually harder that you ever think it's going to be. There's a lot to learn about fertility and conception, and considerations to make about what donor or sperm bank you're going to use. Other questions abound. When should you start trying to get pregnant? How are you going to define your family? What legal advice do you need to make sure your partner is a full parent? And when you do start trying, life splits itself into the inevitable two-week cycles of trying and waiting that could drive any sane woman mad. Even pregnancy itself, that overglorified state of female fullness, is its own roller-coaster ride of changes.

Perhaps you've always wanted to have a child, and after years of thinking about it, you're finally ready to take the plunge. Or it could be that your biological clock just started ticking yesterday and you're all set to educate yourself and then get busy. Maybe you're a single woman, either by choice or circumstance, and you're ready to have a much-longed-for child, bravely and confidently proceeding without a partner. Could be you're with the partner of your dreams and ready to start the family you've always talked about. You may be a straight or bisexual woman fed up with mainstream pregnancy books and looking for more information on how to conceive without a male partner. Whatever the case, whoever you are, the fact that you found this book is a good first step toward realizing your goal of getting pregnant, or being there for someone who is. I welcome all of you to this, the second edition of *The Ultimate Guide to Pregnancy for Lesbians.*

In case you didn't realize it (but I'll bet you did!), there's a tremendous baby boom (or *gayby* boom, in queer lingo) happening among lesbians across the United States, Canada, and the rest of the world. Current statistics estimate the number of children in the United States living with a gay or lesbian parent at between 6 and 14 million. This figure is based on research done in the early 1990s by the National Adoption Information Clearinghouse, a service of the U.S. Administration for Children and Families. One can imagine that the number has grown considerably since then.

A growing acceptance of queer families, greatly increased access to sperm banks and other reproductive technologies, more support services available online, more adoption and surrogacy options for lesbians and gay men, and a noticeable surge in the urge to procreate among younger lesbians are all part of this boom. It is true that women who live in larger urban areas may have more options for services. But with the increased use of the Internet for gathering information and the willingness of sperm banks to ship almost anywhere in the world, there is no reason why almost any lesbian cannot realize her dream of becoming a mother through birth or other means.

This is a pregnancy book, to be sure, and one for a general lesbian readership, concentrating on the biological realities of conceiving and having a low-risk pregnancy and birth. However, I certainly encourage women to explore all options open to them in bringing children into their lives. Lesbians often have so much to give, and are such good, thoughtful parents, that I particularly applaud women who choose nonbiological routes to parenthood like adoption or fostering. Certainly there is no shortage of needy children in the world seeking good homes.

Of course, lesbians choosing to have children is not a new "fad." Indeed, lesbians have always had children, mostly through heterosexual relationships and marriage. Since the 1970s, lesbians have had children through donor insemination, often using the sperm of gay male friends back in the days before AIDS. Today, lesbian-friendly and single-mother-friendly sperm banks abound. Some are even owned by lesbians or gay men, and most offer special guidance to their lesbian clients. Sperm can be shipped internationally in liquid nitrogen tanks, so if you use a sperm bank, your child may have a half sibling or two across the world. Indeed, the only impediments to a lesbian getting pregnant today, aside from her own fertility problems, are the cost and time involved.

According to many sperm banks, the average length of time it takes to become pregnant with frozen sperm is about a year. Of course, we all want to believe that we'll get pregnant on the first attempt, and we all know at least one dyke who tried once on a whim and scored her first time. However, the odds of this are low, and some women never get pregnant, despite years of trying.

But let's start at the beginning, shall we? In this book, you will learn about your body's natural patterns of fertility, which you may never have known even existed. You'll read all about sperm banks and how to pick a donor, how to inseminate at home, and what happens if you do so at a doctor's office or fertility clinic. You'll be guided through the rough months of trying to conceive, gently led through the first stages of pregnancy, given advice on self-care and nutrition, and presented with an honest look at the hormonal and bodily changes you'll go through. Advice and encouragement are a given here—whether you are a single mom or part of a couple. There's even special information included for partners of pregnant women. After all, not only are they supporting their partner's pregnancy, they're going through their own unique changes.

All three trimesters of a healthy pregnancy are covered here in detail, including week-by-week development of the growing baby. I'll help you think about birthing options, guide you through birth's different stages, and I'll even let you in on the realities of your first few tumultuous weeks of motherhood. There are sections on infertility and sex during pregnancy, two topics that most mainstream pregnancy books don't cover. And all of this is written and presented with the deep understanding and empathy of a fellow queer girl mama. May I also add that this book is fun to read, and free of the fear that plagues some other popular pregnancy books?

As someone who has been through this whole process, it is my hope in writing this book that I can provide the information that lesbians are really looking for. When I got pregnant, I was living in San Francisco, the epicenter of the lesbian baby boom. Yet I felt very alone while trying to get pregnant. Why? First, I didn't have a network of other dykes along on the same journey. Second, the mainstream pregnancy books I turned to for conception advice all assumed that their readers had already conceived—and often by accident! The few lesbian parenting books on the market, while well-meaning, were short on the details of conception and long on psychobabble. The first sperm bank I used seemed more concerned with profits than with providing support or accurate information. My friends, none of whom had children or had tried to conceive, hadn't a clue about what I was going through or any idea about how to be supportive. My girlfriend at the time, while mildly encouraging of my idea to get pregnant, was not a supportive partner, and she frequently made me feel like an obsessed freak. There was no wealth of online support in those days for lesbians trying to conceive. It was a lonely and difficult time for me.

During a particularly hard time in my conception journey (and unknowingly, the same month I would actually get pregnant), I wrote an article for *Curve* magazine. This was in the days before glossy gay parenting magazines or websites, and I was dismayed by the lack of information in the queer press about lesbian pregnancy. I approached my friend and *Curve*'s publisher Franco Stevens about running a piece on my frustrations as a dyke trying to conceive. This article, probably the first ever to appear in the mainstream queer press about lesbian pregnancy, was published in *Curve* in March 1998, and the response was overwhelming. Hundreds of women from all over the world wrote me, asking about my quest and offering support for what was to become my very public journey to and through pregnancy. This tremendous outpouring of good wishes from women who'd been in my shoes led me to believe that there was a very real need for a book such as this one. Luckily, the good folks at Cleis Press agreed (and still agree), and what was only a hunch has become a best-selling reality.

It is thus with great pride that I present to you the second edition of *The Ultimate Guide to Pregnancy for Lesbians*. Most of it was written during the summer when I was pregnant with my daughter, Frances, and the realities of what I went through inform every page. For the revised edition, I revisited these sections with the wiser eye of a few years' hindsight.

Also appearing throughout the text are advice and opinions from many experts who spoke exclusively with me to provide information just for you. Chief among them is Kate Kendell, Director of the National Center for Lesbian Rights, who gave me updated legal information for this second edition. Cheers go to Deborah Simone and Anne Semans, who gave me information on pregnancy and birth and sexuality. You'll also get a new and rare behind-the-scenes look at one of the country's pioneering sperm banks—the Sperm Bank of California—with lead health worker Cathy Winks. Both Cathy and Anne are well-known writers on women's and lesbian-specific health and sexuality, and I am delighted to include their voices here. And as always, my thanks to the many lesbians who responded to my calls for what became the real-life quotes you will see scattered throughout this book.

So sit back, relax, and get ready for the ride of your life. Your conception attempts and pregnancy may be very trying at times, but this book will be right there to provide encouragement, as well as to answer the inevitable barrage of questions you're bound to have. Of course, as with any health advice book, the information here should never replace the advice of a licensed health-care practitioner. I wish you all the best on your journey, and when the going gets tough, remember that this book was written by someone who's been in your shoes. And if I could do it, chances are that you can, too!

2

Thinking It Over
and Making a Plan

Deciding to have a child will be the biggest decision you ever make. No matter what else you do during the course of your lifetime—whether it be starting a business, moving across the country, or falling in love—there is nothing so profound as creating a new life. It will rock every preconceived idea you have of what it means to love or live fully in the world. There is so much to consider when planning for a baby, but one fact remains constant no matter what your circumstances: From an abstract idea about "having a baby" will eventually grow a real, live, breathing creature with a personality and will all its own!

Your pregnancy and the birth of your baby will be a fantastic voyage into new, uncharted territory. At times, this trip will be filled with elation; other times it will seem maddeningly full of frustration. And before you even start on this path, you will have many questions to grapple with. These questions include wondering how you'll get pregnant, and whether you'll use a sperm bank or a known donor. Most women begin thinking about pregnancy with a look toward the future, trying to see how a baby will fit into their world. That's a very good place to start.

Among straight women, many a pregnancy is planned with the same care that lesbians bring to the process. But there are also many straight women who conceive by accident and figure things out as they go. On the other hand, any woman, straight or gay, who intentionally conceives without having sex with a man has probably really thought through the decision to parent. Lesbians, in particular, are often very careful advance planners who have given an unusual amount of thought to the process and what it might mean to be a parent. And have no doubt, the work you will do in planning the best time and the best way to have your baby will go far in making you an even more wonderful parent.

Of course, there may not be a perfect time or way to have your baby, and there is no real way to fully prepare for the incredible and often startling changes that having your first baby will bring to your life. Still, some times for conception are preferable to others, based on the status of your health, your age, your work situation, your financial and emotional stability, and the amount of time you have to devote to your baby. Everything in your world, from your relationship to your family, your partner, your finances, your social life, your job, to how you feel about your own bodily and spiritual essence, will be dramatically altered. Before you make a baby you should be very, very sure that you are in a good place in your life and are conscious of the inevitable changes that will occur.

I know this sounds very serious, and it should. A baby is not just a cute bundle we feel biologically driven to create, or a way to fit in with the largely heterosexual world around us. Babies grow up quickly and become children, with their own issues and challenges. Everything must revolve around their needs. Their personalities, school schedules, food preferences, habits, and interests often vary significantly from our own.

You can count on some of the following occurring with a newborn in the house:

- You will get much less sleep, and likely be continually tired
- You will feel different about your body, which may be radically altered by pregnancy and childbirth
- Your hormones will be racing, and you may suffer from postpartum depression
- You may worry more about danger in the world
- Someone else's needs will come first now—and yours likely last
- You may feel isolated, particularly if you are a single mom
- You'll feel cut off from your childless friends and wonder what you have in common with them now
- You may miss your old professional life and feel conflicted about being away from your previous work even if you want to be home with your baby

- You may become frustrated at the relentless and constant care babies require
- Money will become a larger concern as you realize how expensive childrearing is
- Your relationship with your partner will change as you renegotiate life as a family with a child

Now that I have scared you a bit, let me reassure you by telling you that having a baby was the best thing I ever did. Having a child is always a leap of faith, and at some points you just have to jump! Don't get caught up in planning every detail so carefully that you wait unnecessarily, and put off getting pregnant for too long. You may find yourself facing fertility problems if you wait past the age of 35. It is better to tolerate a few unknowns in the larger equation than risk not being able to conceive at all.

If you're like me, you probably always wanted to have a child, and you are willing to cope with any hardships involved to bring a child into your life. And there is so much joy. Not only will you fulfill your dream of having a child by birthing a baby, you will join a worldwide community of mothers by doing so. This community is truly a bonded sisterhood of women, regardless of your sexual orientation. You will also feel a new capacity to love and protect another person, a renewed sense of wonder in life, and possibly a greater concern for larger social issues including the health of the planet.

It's also good to know in advance that the tremendous adjustments of new parenthood do ease up after the first year. Baby boot camp—what I call those first few rough months—will soon give way to a confidence in your own parenting. This will give you greater strength in all your experiences in life. It is a wondrous transformation.

So, again, the best first step you can take when considering parenthood is to realistically assess your own situation and contemplate how a child will fit into your life. I will cover the more nitty-gritty aspects of reproduction, like selecting a sperm donor, in future chapters. But here are some of the biggest areas of concern for women along the pregnancy path, and some points to ponder. Let's start with the state of the lesbian parenting nation, and move into the areas of work, finances, home life, your body and self-care, and your support system. Interspersed with my text throughout the book will be quotes from real women who have walked down this very same path.

The State of the Lesbian Parenting Nation

As I wrote in the last chapter, the number of children being raised in lesbian households is growing. Census 2000, which counted cohabiting gay and lesbian couples nationally for the first time, found children under the age of 18 in one-third of households headed by lesbians. This translates to a rough estimate of as many as 14 million children. The number doesn't even include single parents, lesbians living with men, or any other truly nontraditional parenting combination. Think about it—all those kids being raised by queers! So, unless you live in a tiny town, you won't be the first lesbian parent or family in your neck of the woods. If you are, it may be a rough journey as people around you adapt to your family. But most dykes starting families find themselves in good company as the queer baby boom rages on.

There are special websites and magazines just for us, and organizations like the Family Pride Coalition that exist solely to support glbtq families. There are queer family cruises, gay "family weeks" in queer enclaves like Provincetown that attract more than 500 families, and the Michigan Womyn's Music Festival has a booming family camp area—complete with wonderful, free childcare. Lesbian families are common in cities like New York and San Francisco, and they exist across every state and province. It's a great time to be a lesbian mom. And since I believe that most queer parents are extremely good at raising their children, and their kids are so wanted and well loved, I have no doubt that this quiet revolution in parenting is changing the very face of the country.

Are Lesbian Parents Great Parents?

I think so. The amount of planning that goes into creating our children, and the thoughtfulness that we bring to this decision, and subsequently to our parenting, make us generally exceptional parents. Furthermore, many of us wait to have our kids till our thirties and forties, when we have matured enough to deal calmly with most of the challenges of parenthood. Of course, I am generalizing here. I don't like every dyke mom I meet, nor do I think all lesbians should be parents. Indeed, I know some very irritating lesbian parents with equally bratty children, but I never felt that their children were less than well cared for and adored. I really believe that if more straight people planned their families as carefully as most lesbians, and parented in as thoughtful a way, there would be many more happy, healthy children in the world.

Redefining Family Structures

Most lesbians have babies while in relationships with other women. Some go it solo. There are other combinations that work for some single women—including coparenting with a gay man, with a gay male couple, or sharing custody with a straight man or another woman. Lesbian couples sometimes find coparenting with a male couple works well, especially if one of the men is the biological father. Be careful in your utopian family planning, however. The more people involved in a parenting situation, the higher the odds that conflicts will arise. As more and more lesbian couples coparent with gay male couples, it's imperative that good communication and proper legal preparation set the stage for the birth of any new family.

If you feel you would like to parent, but cannot or do not want to do it alone or in a couple, there are groups that can connect gay men and lesbians looking to parent together. There is even an online "conception connection" registry that will link lesbian, gay, bisexual and transgendered folks who want to have biological children with a previously unknown partner. See the resources section for details.

What about the Kids?

There are absolutely no statistics that prove that kids raised by lesbians are much different from those raised by straight folk. In fact, recent studies affirm our fitness in parenting. Even Dr. Spock has weighed in on the issue. In an online column, Spock, or whoever now writes as Spock, stated that our children are comparable to all other children in their mental health, are as likely to be heterosexual as children raised in straight families, and are less likely to suffer sexual abuse in the home (since straight men are the biggest perpetrators of abuse); they also grow up more tolerant of differences in others. Indeed, I happen to believe that our children are more empathetic, worldly, and adaptable than most children. Compared to children raised in straight and narrow-minded families, our kids know that life holds more options. In other words, our kids fare just as well as most children, and probably even better.

Will My Kids Be Teased?

Probably. But accept that and move on. Every kid is teased for something, and you have a few years to worry about it before it happens from
the time you conceive. Do straight people worry that they'll produce a
child who'll get teased about having flaming red hair or unusually big
feet? Do they worry about their very short, or very tall, or deaf, or biracial child getting teased, and wonder how that child will fit in with his or
her peers? Of course, but they understand that guiding their children
through the difficulties of growing up in a different household is part of
the job of parenting.

The Working Mom

Are you self-employed? Work part-time? Hold a demanding full-time
job? If you work full-time, is there any possibility of flextime? Does your
company offer maternity leave? "Paternity," or new parental leave, for
your partner? How much time? Can you work part-time during the latter
part of your pregnancy if you need to cut back? How do you see your
work life changing after you have a baby? Are you planning to go back to
work? When? Can you afford to work part-time? Will you want to
work at all? If you have a partner, will she support the household while
you take a year or more off? Is her job stable? Does she want to stay
home with the baby while you go back to work in a few months? If you're
self-employed, do you have someone lined up to take over some of your
clients? If you own or run a business, do you have an assistant poised to
step in for an indeterminate time? Can you take your baby to work with
you? Are you a student, and your work is school? How will having a baby
affect your studies and your goals for finishing a degree? Are you setting
all your plans in stone, or are you allowing yourself the flexibility to
change your mind after the baby is actually here?

Work takes up a huge chunk of our adult lives and is often a satisfying
part of our self-identity. For those who are not independently wealthy or
supported full-time by a lover or parents, work is also how we support
ourselves and our children. While many women work right through their
pregnancies and rebound quickly after their baby's birth, most will need
to curtail their working hours before the birth and slow down after their
baby arrives. Growing a baby is hard work. It will make you tired and probably increasingly uncomfortable, grouchy, and even a bit brain-muddled.

By my own seventh month of pregnancy, I had to really cut back on the amount of time I spent in the small business I owned. I was fortunate to be my own boss; I came back to work slowly, sometimes bringing my baby with me, sometimes hiring a babysitter. When my daughter turned a year old, she started going to childcare four days a week, and that's when I began to feel that my entry back into the world of work was gearing back up. Even then, I didn't work a 9-to-5 job till she turned 5 years old, in part because I had previously had the luxury of setting my own hours in my own business, and because it was just too exhausting to work full-time. Also, I wanted to spend a lot of time with my daughter while she was young, enjoying lazy afternoons at the playground or going to art and swim classes together. Those precious early years speed by quickly indeed; I'm glad I was around to enjoy them.

Maternity Leave

Both our employers were spectacular about our maternity leaves. I saved up my vacation time and got three months paid leave. My partner got about the same and then started back up at work part-time. We are both out at our jobs, and we had no problems at all with discrimination about this. —Pam

Most larger companies have well-defined policies about maternity leave. Some have wonderful benefits, some don't. Find out what these are, well in advance of becoming pregnant. If you can receive paid maternity leave, plan to take full advantage of what is offered, even if you're not sure you'll need it or even want to return to your job. You can always go back to work early, or change your mind about working at all. Recovering from childbirth can take longer than you'd imagine, and it's time well spent in bonding with your baby. If you are eligible only for vacation time, start saving up the hours. If you get unpaid leave, start setting aside money. If you work for a smaller company, there may be less chance of receiving benefits and more pressure to return or have your job filled by someone else. On the other hand, both large and small companies are capable of creating progressive policies that encourage a realistic balance of family and work lives. If you're lucky, you'll also work for an employer that encourages breastfeeding (so you can take the time to pump at work) and may even have onsite day care. If day care is provided, make sure you register early—there is often a long waiting list.

If You're Self-Employed

I am self-employed and work from home. I had to start working a week after the baby was born. In a way this was easy, but in another very tiring. But I had no other choice financially....

—Sage

If you are self-employed, you won't have a boss breathing down your neck, but you may not be able to take as much of a break after the baby is born. Will you close up shop for a few weeks? Or will things run smoothly in your absence with trusted employees taking up the slack? If you run a one-person business, you may want to consider bringing a part-time person on board so they will be trained when you become pregnant. If you work at home, can you swap childcare with another home-based mom so you can work baby-free a few hours a day? If you own a store, will it be possible for you to bring your baby to work with you? I took Frances to the bookstore I owned for the first few months of her life, but by five months she was bored and wiggly and ready for a part-time babysitter who could concentrate solely on her—and not on the store's customers! Babies grow up very quickly, and it will be too hard to focus on your clients if the baby is crying because she's hungry, pulling items off the store's shelves, or about to run out the door of your business! Having your baby at work with you full-time is a nice ideal, but in all honesty, it's not very practical or productive beyond the first few months.

Partners and Parental Leave

As more companies in North America become family friendly, many are issuing paternity leave or leave for same-sex partners in the event of a birth or adoption of a baby. This can range from a few days to several months. To negotiate longer leaves, you may have to use accumulated vacation or sick time. I strongly recommend that partners take as much time as they can after the baby is born. The birth mother will need you, and likely you will want to be there for both her and the baby. It will be utterly exhausting to try to hold down a full-time job, run the house, fully participate in parenting, and care for your hormonally crashing, lactating partner. Give yourself a break and use as much parental leave as you can get. You will thank me—and your partner will thank you—for this advice.

Finances

Like it or not, it's very expensive to raise a child. Even if you plan to breastfeed and resist buying lots of "baby stuff," there are plenty of expenses that you won't anticipate until they come up. And the cost of childcare can be the biggest case of sticker shock you ever experience as a parent! Figure that childcare alone will cost you between $40 and $60 a day for most home day-care or group-care facilities. That's up to $300 a week, or $1,200 a month. A nanny in urban areas will cost $15 to $20 an hour. True, some people never use day care, or are able to raise children without much financial planning. The more sensible scenario is to do some advance preparation. Here are some basic tips to help get your prebaby finances in order.

Pay Off Your Debt

If you are seriously in debt, it's wise to clear up as much of it as possible before you start trying to conceive. In particular, I'm thinking of the consumer debt that plagues so many of us. Not only is the interest rate a killer—the last thing you need is creditors knocking on your door while you are pregnant. If your credit score or debt load is bad, you may find it harder, later on, to buy a much-needed larger home or even find a better rental. Not to mention that if your credit cards are maxed out, those late-night trips to buy diapers will be extremely stressful!

Save for Conception and Childbirth

It can cost thousands of dollars to conceive and have your baby. Count on saving at least $5,000 to get pregnant, and a few thousand more for either a complication-free vaginal home birth or regular hospital birth. These costs can easily double or triple if you take longer than expected to get pregnant. If you have health insurance, find out how much of your conception services may be covered, and what percentage of the cost of your pre- and postnatal care. You might also ask about coverage for infertility treatments, since these also get very pricey. Now would be the time to change health plans if you need to, or get health insurance if you lack it. Complications, such as needing a caesarean section or having a premature baby who needs hospitalization, can send these costs into the stratosphere for the uninsured.

Postbaby Savings

Save some money for after the baby arrives. Plan to have enough for a few months' rent and utilities stashed aside. You may decide not to go back to work; your partner may decide to stay home too; you will need to buy lots of supplies like diapers and baby swings and car seats; and you may decide to use paid help, such as a doula (a woman who helps a mother before, during, and just after childbirth). This is just not the time to be financially strapped.

Home Life

One of the best gifts you can give your child is a happy, stable home life. I say this regardless of whether you are single or in a coupled relationship. Are you truly ready to welcome another person—someone for whom you will have complete responsibility—into your family? Are you done with your hard-core partying? Are you living in a place that seems fit for a child? Are you prepared to feel the pull of the mainstream as you parent in a largely heterosexual world? Have you worked out some of those pesky personal issues that plague us all? Are you feeling in control of your life and the direction it's heading? Good! Now look around you.

Living with Roommates

Do you live with roommates? Do you expect them to play any part in your child's life? Are they fit to do so? Do they already have children? Will their children be excited and understanding about the changes another baby in the household will bring? Are the adult members likely to anticipate your pregnancy with glee or dread? Does anyone in the household have behaviors or addictions that could prove dangerous to a newborn? These are among the questions you will need to ask yourself, and issues you should examine carefully, if you live in a shared-housing situation.

If you live with roommates, you should be honest with them about your plans to conceive. If they seem less than enthusiastic or are in any way unfit to live with a young child, you might want to find a new dwelling, or ask them to. Keep in mind that this may cause irrevocable damage to a friendship. I had to ask a much-loved old friend to move out of my house when Frances was about a year old. He had only lived with us for a few months when I realized his drinking problem was back, and worsening, and leading to occasionally dangerous behaviors. The room-mate relationship had to end, and unfortunately so did the friendship. As a mother, you will need to put the best interests and safety of your child first, whatever the costs.

Choosing to Live Alone

If you are unpartnered, or just choose to live alone, you can set up the kind of home you want for yourself and your baby. Just make sure to line up enough support for yourself after the baby is born. This support includes making sure someone is available to help you cook and clean during the first few weeks, offer knowledge and encouragement for breastfeeding, give you occasional breaks to shower and go for a short walk, and lend a kind ear as you talk about the transition to new moth-erhood. There will be more information and ideas later in the book about support for single moms.

Living with Girlfriends

There's a joke circulating around the lesbian community that goes some-thing like this: "What does a lesbian bring to a first date? A U-Haul. What does she bring to the second? A turkey baster." Well, a turkey baster is certainly the wrong tool for the job of insemination, but you get the gist of the joke. Baby-making has become a popular lesbian pastime. But it's not anything to rush into.

If you are in a long-term, committed relationship with another woman and are planning to raise a child together, you are definitely in the majority of my readership. If yours is a stable relationship and you have been together a few years, and this is a dream you both share, then you are in a good position to begin planning a family. However, if the relationship is new, unstable, violent, or one that causes you any doubt, it would be best to do some more soul-searching before you birth a child. Don't make the mistake so many straight couples make: having a child to "save" or even define the relationship. You could be setting yourself up for nasty custody battles down the road.

Think about whether you really need a partner to become pregnant or raise a child. I have seen many single dykes, desperate to have a child, scout around to find a partner just so they can go ahead with baby-making. True, it's more affordable and logistically easier with two adults. However, a girlfriend gotten does not a perfect relationship—or a proper parent—make. My last word on this is to be careful: As more dykes have children together, more custody cases involving the children of lesbian moms are heading to court.

If, however, you've been with someone long-term and you've soul-searched together enough to know what it means to have, and raise, a child together, then you're ready to proceed—as the loving team that you are.

In some couples, both women may relish the thought of biologically carrying a child. How can this be worked out? Perhaps you will both decide to give birth, a few years apart. The older partner, or the one who feels most strongly about birthing, could try first. Some women actually try at the same time, and end up pregnant together. I know couples who have done this, and they all say it is difficult. With both women feeling hormonal and in need of support, it can make for a very rocky nine months. And then, both will be feeling exhausted and postpartum at the same time, and there will be two newborns in the house to care for. It's like having twins, but even more exhausting.

Other couples find the question of who will carry the baby a nonissue, because one woman is more prone to seek pregnancy. The other will happily coparent as the other mom, or, in the case of a butch or tranny partner, as the dyke daddy or tranny pop. However, it is not always the more femme partner who chooses to birth a baby. Although not as frequently, butch women also make the decision to get pregnant, and FTMs who still have their female reproductive organs are also capable of getting pregnant and giving birth. This book is for all of you.

Assessing Your Support System

If You Are Single

Some women, myself included, want to be single mothers. Usually we're an independent lot, financially stable, maybe emotionally wary, and our biological clocks are ticking. One of the best things about being a single mom is the freedom to make decisions for your child. I don't have to endlessly process every issue and decision with a partner, or compromise on my parenting beliefs to keep the peace. If I say it's okay for Frances to have a Popsicle at the playground before dinner, no partner is going to scold me later. If I want to move cross-country or to Mexico with Frances, no one can stop me. In a single-parent family, there is often less or no competition for the mom's attention from other adults. As a result, single parents and their children are often very close. These are just a few of the things that are good about single parenting.

A large contingent of single straight women are "single mothers by choice." This is much less common in the lesbian community. Why? Part of it may be due to the economic costs of conceiving and raising a child, or just that the two-mommy family most closely resembles the heteronormative nuclear family many of us grew up with. Many people still think that having two parents, regardless of their gender or the strength of their relationship, is preferable to single parenting.

If you are thinking about single parenting, you should know that it will be tough. This I say from personal experience and the experience of other single moms I've talked to. We all agree, there are two major factors that will help keep you sane: having an adequate support system and having adequate financial means. Without the proper cash flow, single parenting turns dreary very fast. You will struggle just to make ends meet and pay the babysitter, and you can forget about vacations, movies, and the occasional margarita! To avoid this plight, make sure your financial house is in order before you conceive, reconsider the line of work you do if necessary, and look carefully at the costs of childcare where you live. Remember, short of babysitting co-ops or the goodwill of family, if you are not watching your baby, you will be paying someone else to do it.

Could You Parent a Special-Needs Child?

Along with all the considerations you'll be making about having a baby, you should think about whether you're prepared to parent a special-needs child. If your genetic testing reveals a likelihood of Down syndrome, what are you likely to feel, or do? If very serious birth defects are detected during genetic testing, would you carry the child to term? How do you feel about abortion in such circumstances? This is a conversation you should have with yourself, and with your partner if you're coupled, before you decide to conceive a child.

A strong support system is a lifesaver for a single parent, and proper planning can help create one. While pregnant, you will need the support of childless friends as well as other mamas to talk to and help you get ready for the baby. Taking care of a baby is often overwhelming, especially when you and your baby are alone for extended periods. The needs of a baby are so intense that you can go nuts giving continually without a break for your own needs—even if it's just to bathe or to take a five-minute walk alone. It is simply too much to expect that you can truly do it all yourself, no matter how much you want a child. You need to have one or two trusted friends you can call who will understand how relentless the task of mothering is, and who will take the baby for an hour when you need a break.

The best time to start priming friends for becoming aunties is even before conception. Let friends know you are going to attempt to get pregnant. Talk to them about what this will mean for you, and ask them if they would like to participate in the baby's life. Some friends will be excited, others lukewarm to the idea, and still others clearly uninterested. Many will change their minds about how they feel, one way or another, over the course of your pregnancy. I think that if you can find even two or three people to provide ongoing auntie care for your growing child, or to be someone you can talk to honestly about mothering, you are doing really well. Out of a circle of about ten good friends I had hoped would be involved in my daughter's life, only two really stepped up and stayed involved. A few who I thought would be especially interested disappeared into the drama of their own lives, which I found disappointing.

After you have your baby, you may find that your biggest support will come from other single moms—often straight women you didn't know before the birth of your child, or theirs. Try to find an online bulletin board for single mothers or single mothers-to-be. (See the resources section.) These boards are full of extremely supportive women who are also very knowledgeable about conception and pregnancy. Keep your ears open at work and among friends for news of any other woman who is beginning her parenting journey solo, or who has just had a child. Get her phone number and call her. She may well become one of your most trusted friends.

Keeping your eyes open for a good childcare provider even before the baby is born will help you ease into a comfortable relationship with your first babysitter. In fact, as a single mom, you would do well to visit childcare centers or home day cares and get onto waiting lists as needed. Usually the best providers and centers have at least a one-year waiting list, and they often let you save a slot when you conceive. It will be one less thing to worry about when you have a newborn.

If You Are Coupled

If you are in a coupled relationship and are planning to raise a child together, you will have one another to lean on during the trying times of conception and pregnancy. Even so, it will not be enough support. Babies are more work than you can plan for and may overwhelm even the best-prepared couples. Especially in the difficult early months, it is best to have established a support system of people who can at least help with cooking and cleaning. Luxuries like childcare for an occasional meal out together will go far toward maintaining some sanity in your lives and stability in your relationship. Try to befriend other couples you like who are also expecting or trying to conceive. You'll have a great network of friends once your baby arrives, and other parents to trade babysitting with.

Ways to meet other couples include scanning a gay center's bulletin board, logging onto a lesbian parenting website, or contacting a lesbian midwife. You could even start a group for lesbian moms if one doesn't exist in your area. It will be reassuring to meet other women who are going through the same things you are. If you maintain friendships with childless friends and you are lucky enough to have supportive family nearby, encourage these folks to be invested in your growing family. It will mean a wider world for your child to grow into, and free childcare for you and your partner later! You will also find that you now have more in common with straight couples trying to conceive than with the general, nonparenting lesbian community. The journey of the lesbian couple into child-rearing is unique, and as a couple you will need unique support and respect for the wonderful journey you are on together.

A Special Note to Younger Women

The biological urge to have a baby can be very strong in young women, and I know several young lesbians who have chosen to parent. Your late teens and your twenties are a prime time for your body to bear a child. Your reproductive system is healthy, your fertility is high, and you have ample energy for pregnancy, childbirth, and parenting. However, I urge caution. Your urge to parent will not go away, and you will still be fertile in your late twenties and early thirties. In the meantime, finish school. Find a career path. Establish yourself in a healthy environment and create a base of adult friends who will provide emotional support for this journey. Ensure your partnership is a solid one. Make sure your finances reflect your commitment to parenting. Travel. Party. Entertain. Finish some of the lifework you're meant to do before the hard work of parenting begins. I guarantee all this will make you a better, more mature parent when you do begin your parenting journey.

Legal Protections for Lesbian Families

The National Center for Lesbian Rights is there to assist lesbians in the legal planning of their future families. In an interview, NCLR Director Kate Kendell said it is "imperative that you seek the advice of a local attorney competent in how family law operates in your state" when considering parenting with another person. The best way to find such an attorney, she said, is by word of mouth from other local lesbians. If you don't know anyone who can make referrals, the NCLR will give you the names of some attorneys in your state who may be knowledgeable.

Kendell urges couples contemplating coparenting to talk deeply about every issue of parenting and draw up legal agreements. She reminds readers that such documents are not often legally upheld in court as enforceable. However, she says, "The process of creating such a document with purposeful attention will help clarify many issues in case of crisis later on." Women who live in states and provinces where domestic partnerships or marriage are available to them will be a step ahead in legally protecting their families. In fact, in California, because of a law that went into effect in 2005, a child born to registered domestic partners is now considered legally the child of both parents! This means both

> *Prior to inseminating, all women should see a lawyer to discuss issues about known versus unknown donors, second-partner adoptions, and advice with respect to their role and involvement as parents.*
>
> —Kate Kendell, Director, National Center for Lesbian Rights

parents can be named on the child's birth certificate, and both are responsible financially for the child. Expect the rest of the country to follow suit, very slowly but also very surely. In the meantime, see a competent attorney, and check the NCLR website for updates on the status of family law in your area: www.nclrights.org.

Safer Sex Starts Now

Before you begin trying to conceive is the perfect time to review your safer-sex practices. Many sexually transmitted diseases, such as HIV, chlamydia, and herpes, can be passed along to the fetus or can complicate pregnancy. Naturally, you will get a complete gynecological checkup, including tests for HIV, hepatitis B and C, chlamydia, gonorrhea, syphilis, herpes, and so on. While you are trying to get pregnant, be extra vigilant about your sexual health. If you and your girlfriend have sex only with each other and have tested negative for HIV and other STIs, your safer-sex requirements are much simplified. Here are a few guidelines to keep in mind:

- Remember that your girlfriend needs to keep up her gynecological care, too. Fluid-bonding (sharing bodily fluids only with a primary partner; using latex and other barriers with any other partners) works only if you both commit to good health practices. A pesky vaginal infection can be transmitted through oral sex.
- Keep your toys clean. Use condoms on dildos and vibrators to prevent sharing of vaginal infections.
- Do not allow anal bacteria access to the vagina. After anal sex and before vaginal sex, wash your hands, rinse your mouth, discard that latex glove or condom, and clean your toys.
- Do not use oil-based lubricants (like Crisco, Vaseline, or baby oil) for vaginal penetration. Oil-based lube does not rinse out of the vagina very easily and thus provides a great breeding ground for vaginal infections. Use water-based lubes instead.
- If you have more than one sex partner, or if you or your partner may have been exposed to an STI, it's time to make some decisions about safer-sex practices. Unprotected sex between women—particularly cunnilingus, and particularly during menstruation—*can* transmit STIs. Educate yourself, talk with your girlfriend(s), and make informed decisions for your health.

Toxoplasmosis

Toxoplasmosis is a disease that can cause birth defects in the baby if the mother is infected during pregnancy. It is contracted from contact with the feces of cats that have eaten infected mice. If you already have antibodies to the *Toxoplasma* pathogen before you get pregnant, you can't pass the disease to your fetus. But if you test negative, you must be extremely careful changing your cat's litter box while you are pregnant. Have someone else do it, or wear disposable rubber gloves each time you change the box. I kept a box of gloves on a table right next to the litter box so I wouldn't forget. Try to keep the litter box as clean as you can to avoid inhaling the fumes of feces.

Health Tests You Will Need Before You Conceive

Even before you start inseminating, eat like a queen, use only purified water, get in the habit of exercising regularly, and quit smoking. It really isn't too early to prepare the future baby-building machine for the most wholesome environment you can give that little one. —Stephanie

On my first visit to an RE, I had an ultrasound, and lots of blood drawn for a whole array of tests. The bloodwork was to check my hormonal levels and for STDs. My RE recommended an HSG test to see if my tubes were blocked, and I was given a routine breast exam. If you have insurance, these tests are highly recommended. IUI is an expensive trip. It is better to make sure you are okay before you begin. —Diana

Now is the time to see what condition your body is in to grow a baby. While you may feel totally healthy and have no symptoms of illness, most fertility clinics and sperm banks will ask that you have a variety of health tests before you begin trying to conceive. *Allow two months before you actually start trying to get pregnant to have these tests and get the results. If you don't, you may be disappointed if the test or treatment process drags on and you can't begin trying to conceive when you were planning to.*

It can be time-consuming and expensive, but I suggest you get all the recommended tests. Typically, you may be required to receive Pap and chlamydia smears, blood work for HIV, HTLV-1, CMV, syphilis, rubella, toxoplasmosis (see sidebar on page 23), Tay-Sachs disease (a fairly rare genetic disease among some Jews), and sickle-cell anemia, if you are African American. My sperm bank even insisted I receive a test for something called mycoureaplasma, a low-grade infection of the reproductive tract, which many women have without realizing it. It is suspected of causing miscarriage and can prevent you from getting pregnant. I scoffed at taking that one in particular, and guess what—I tested positive for it. Luckily, a small dose of antibiotics cleared it from my system. Because of my experience, I would urge you to ask for this test even if your doctor doesn't require it. If you have a history of endometriosis, you will want to have a test to see if your fallopian tubes are viable. You could need laparoscopic surgery to unblock the tubes and get rid of any adhesions or remaining endometriosis.

Conditions for Concern

> *In some ways, I think having a high risk pregnancy had its real advantages. We saw the doctor frequently and never went long without a question being answered. In the end, I suspect that I had a healthier pregnancy than many women. —Janet*

If you think you may be a candidate for a high-risk pregnancy because of existing health problems, you should consult a doctor or other trusted health-care professional before you begin to inseminate. Diabetes, which came up often among women I talked to in researching this book, is a good example of a condition you will need to monitor closely during pregnancy. Other health issues to talk to your provider about include past ectopic pregnancies, miscarriages, and abortions. If you are over 40 years old, you will be told that not only might you have a harder time conceiving, you also have a greater risk of miscarriage and of having a baby born with Down syndrome.

While some women go into pregnancy knowing they could have difficulties, don't forget that any pregnancy can become a high-risk one. Conditions such as placenta previa, where the placenta blocks the cervix, or preeclampsia, where the woman develops high blood pressure, can strike any woman during her pregnancy. With careful monitoring, however, most such conditions don't interfere with a woman's ability to carry her baby to term.

> *Friends told us that pregnancy with a condition like diabetes is like the normal experience of pregnancy times ten. We were very dependent on a competent and up-to-date medical team who supported our decision to get pregnant. We were so glad that we had each other and that our team respected our decisions.*
> —Nicca

> *I have a history of diabetes and although I was very healthy at the time I got pregnant, I fully expected gestational diabetes. At eighteen weeks, that diagnosis was confirmed.* —Yvonne

> *I think being an older mom actually was easier for me. Because I'm in my forties, I'm more educated about how the medical system works and was better able to advocate for myself. I eat well, don't drink anymore, and take really good care of myself, which is more than I can say about how I lived in my twenties and thirties. Although it took me over a year to get pregnant, I had few complications and had an easy delivery.* —Joanne

If you live with a condition such as diabetes, talk to other women with a similar experience. Find a doctor who believes in your ability to have a normal pregnancy, with as little intervention as possible. If you are over 40, consider joining an online group to share information with other older moms.

Before you begin trying to conceive, talk to your doctor about any prescription medicines you are taking and decide whether you might be able to go off them for the duration of your pregnancy.

Disability

Many types of physical conditions are labeled "disabilities." These include being hearing impaired or blind, using a wheelchair, having severe asthma, a bad back, or chronic fatigue. Most disabilities are not passed genetically to unborn children. However, if you are planning to become pregnant, you may want to see a genetic counselor to discuss any risks that may be involved in your pregnancy and whether your children might inherit your condition, whatever it may be. Find a supportive midwife or doctor who will be honest and not condescending to you about any risks.

If you have a disability, it's imperative that you organize your household well beforehand and line up lots of extra support for after the baby's birth if you think you'll need it. If you can, plan on extra time to recover from your delivery and get used to the demands of parenthood. It's likely that there will be people who won't understand your desire to become pregnant, or who will assume that you will be unable to cope with a child once it is born. While it's not your job to educate everyone, you should be prepared for questions that come your way concerning your disability during your pregnancy. You may find that people express strong opinions about you even trying to become pregnant. The best form of support for disabled women is to talk with other disabled women who have successfully become pregnant and are parenting children. While local support groups can provide camaraderie, Internet chat groups will likely be easier to participate in if you have a disability that keeps you closer to home.

The Weight Issue

> I was overweight by about fifty pounds when I got pregnant. The doctor didn't seem to think it would impede conception or cause undue stress during pregnancy or birth. I did not develop gestational diabetes, hypertension, or any other medical problem other than sciatica (leg pain radiating from the lower back). But I still advocate getting as much excess weight off as possible before getting pregnant, because complications can result. I was just extremely lucky! —Roberta

Many doctors tell larger-sized women they need to lose weight before conceiving. It is true that obesity can lead to certain health problems, such as diabetes or hypertension. Pregnancy, with the additional work your body must do, and the extra pounds you will put on, can be a lot to handle physically. So losing weight can make your pregnancy easier and help you avoid further complications. However, there is no reason for most women who are slightly or moderately overweight to lose weight in order to conceive or bear children. If you are overweight but in good health and spirits, and you find that your doctor discourages your efforts to become pregnant, you may want to seek a different health-care practitioner. The best thing to remember is to be as fit as you can before getting pregnant. This holds true for women of ALL sizes. A book I recommend is *Carrying a Little Extra: A Guide to Healthy Pregnancy for the Plus-Size Woman*, by Paula Bernstein, Marlene Clark, and Netty Levine.

Deciding to Have a Second Child

If you're already an experienced parent and considering a second or even a third child, more power to you. Although it adds to the chaos factor and to the family finances, having more than one child will be the ideal for many parents. The good news is that you're already a pro at what you're doing by the time you decide to have a second child. Ever hear how "easy" second children are? While some of them may be temperamentally easier, a large part of the effect is probably due to parental experience. Coupled life has already adapted to become family life, and the second child just kind of goes along with the family flow. Although this book is designed primarily for first-time parents, those considering expanding their families will find it useful as well. Wherever possible in the text I have included information and references for those who are already parents. Keep in mind that secondary infertility, where it's much harder for a woman to conceive the second time around, can also strike lesbian families.

The Long and Winding Road Ahead

Despite all the stories you may have heard from other women about what it means to be pregnant or have a baby, your own experience will be completely different. For lesbians, getting pregnant is not so much a quick decision as a long and winding road—fraught with detours and potholes, yet offering the occasional stunning vista. Consider this woman's story:

> *My partner of fifteen years and I have been in the process of becoming moms for five years. We've been through her not wanting to be a mom, moving through that process, coming out to her parents about wanting to be moms, working with a known donor and developing a contract, meeting with a lawyer and two*

different counselors to make it work, that not working, advertising and meeting other potential known donors, working with a gay male couple and developing a contract, that not working, deciding to go the anonymous donor route, me losing my job, trying home-based insemination for six months, finding a job, going with an IUI in the doctor's office, getting pregnant, miscarrying at twelve weeks, not being able to get pregnant again, then going the infertility route with Clomid and facing the possibility of having my eggs harvested if it doesn't work this way! How did it get so complicated? —Sarah

So, there's a lot more to this pregnancy stuff than meets the eye. You may decide that you aren't really ready to go through with all this yet. Or that you're not really sure you want to carry a baby and want to consider adoption instead. Or you may be even more determined to try to get pregnant—immediately! Only you can decide if you're ready to be a mother, and it's a big decision to make. After all, it is the single biggest, most life-altering decision you will ever make. For further reading on deciding whether to become a mom, I recommend Cheri Pies's *Considering Parenthood*. It is a bit outdated as a text but still an excellent first book to help you decide whether motherhood is really for you.

If you do decide you're ready to begin, you'll embark on a wondrous journey to bring a new baby into the world. I'm so pleased you've chosen this book to help guide you. Now let's begin....

Getting Started—
Now the Fun Really Begins!

Now the fun begins! You've had all your health tests, you've probably thought about donor choices, and you're raring to start trying to get pregnant. But please read this chapter, even if you think you just want to get started tomorrow on the whole process. The more you learn now, the smoother it will all go later. And you'll have received a great education about how your body works—a wonderful prelude to all the changes you'll learn about during your pregnancy. Even if you find just a few pieces of information here that you end up using, it'll be worth it.

On Actually Trying to Get Pregnant

> *So many heterosexual pregnancies seem to happen by accident. But being a lesbian, I have spent years getting to this point. Thinking and wondering and thinking some more. And now the time has come to begin to try.... —Iris*

If you're like many lesbians and have never been sexually active with men, fertility issues will be a brave new world to you. If you're like me and spent your teenage years trying *not* to get pregnant with your male partners, you still may not know a lot about how your body actually works. We're not taught much useful information about our bodies as young women. Probably no one has ever explained fertile mucus to you, or what happens when you ovulate. If you've never been pregnant, you may not even believe your body is capable of becoming so. Now, suddenly, after years of being with women and giving nary a thought to birth control, conception, or pregnancy, here you are, wanting to get pregnant and not knowing where to start. It's frightening to start paying out lots of money without knowing if the process will even work. But learning to trust your body, understanding how conception happens, and knowing how you can maximize your chances of its happening are empowering first steps on the path to parenthood.

What Happens During Conception

The Mystery of Ovulation

Consider this your basic course in conception—Conception 101. How does that one little sperm meet that ripe and ready egg, anyway? It's a miraculous process worthy of sonnets, but we'll be brief and factual here. During each cycle, if you are ovulating regularly, your body is ready for pregnancy. Shortly after you finish your period, about 15 eggs, each in its own follicle, start to mature in your ovaries. One will eventually burst through the ovarian wall while the rest disintegrate, unless multiple ovulation, which is responsible for multiple births, occurs. This process is called *ovulation,* and it usually occurs around the middle, or day 14, of a typical 28-day cycle.

If you want to get more detailed, know that the first half of your cycle is called the *follicular phase*. This is the phase when your body is busy preparing the next batch of eggs for fertilization. The follicles in which the eggs are encased mature until one lucky egg (or that egg and its companions) is released. What is difficult is trying to determine *when* that egg will be ready, and therefore when to inseminate. This is because the race to release an egg begins at different times in different women, and even varies from cycle to cycle in the same woman.

The follicular phase of your cycle lasts from the day you get your period until ovulation, whenever that occurs. This can be anywhere from ten to more that twenty days. The amount of estrogen in your body peaks at the point just before the egg is released, and this surge of what is called the *luteinizing hormone* is what ovulation predictor kits monitor. Many women prefer to inseminate a day or so *after* seeing the surge.

The second phase of your cycle, which is called the *luteal phase*, lasts from ovulation until the last day before the start of your next period. This is usually from 12 to 16 days, and almost always 14 days. So, when you are learning to track ovulation, a more accurate way of judging your timing is to remember that it occurs about 14 days *before* the start of your *next* period. Of course, though many books and many doctors refer to the typical 28-day cycle, a significant percentage of women do not have 28-day cycles. Anything from 20 to 40 days is normal, and some women menstruate or ovulate only once every several months. You can see how this variation is critical to any calculations about when ovulation, and therefore insemination, takes place.

Once the egg bursts through the ovarian wall, it is sucked up, often in less than half an hour, by the nearby fallopian tube, where it will remain alive for 6 to 24 hours, awaiting fertilization. Your best chances of conception, some believe, occur if the sperm are already present in the outer fallopian tube, waiting for the egg. In other words, your chances of getting pregnant may increase if you inseminate right before ovulation, so the sperm are ready, but as close to ovulation as possible, so they haven't died off yet. There is debate about this among fertility experts, however. Some believe you should inseminate before ovulation, at the time of your surge or just afterward. Others now recommend inseminating immediately (within hours) after ovulation—which is how I got pregnant. You will have to decide for yourself which makes the most sense to you. Or better yet, combine the two approaches for maximum potential. Try an at-home insemination first, right before your surge—and then try again a day or two later, perhaps with an IUI (intrauterine insemination) at a clinic. Make the most of the technological advances, and the varying opinions, available to you.

Sperm freshly ejaculated can survive for up to five days inside a woman, though three days is more common. Women who use fresh sperm therefore have a larger window of time during which they can ovulate and their donor's sperm can meet the egg. Thus, women who inseminate with fresh sperm often get pregnant with fewer attempts than women using frozen sperm.

The shorter life span of frozen sperm—only one or two days—means that your timing is absolutely critical. When you inseminate at home with frozen sperm, the sperm must make an arduous journey through the fertile cervical mucus, up through the vagina, into the cervix, and on toward the egg. This can take about five hours of the egg's life span of 24 hours—a big chunk of time! There's a lot less time for the sperm to find the egg inside the woman's body. A process called *intrauterine insemination* cuts the travel time of the sperm by placing them right in the cervix or uterus, rather than in the vagina. Think of intrauterine insemination as a kind of Head Start program for the sperm.

When Sperm Meets Egg

Any sperm that do meet the egg are generally among the hardiest and best swimmers of that particular ejaculate. We tend to think of a lone sperm winning the marathon of the egg hunt. Realistically, however, there are millions of sperm inside an inseminating woman, most of which get lost, spin in circles, or are simply immobile. Usually, one small group of the strongest and fastest swimmers remain on course, and they all race together to find and penetrate the waiting egg. When one sperm does break through the outer membrane of the egg, it is immediately drawn into the egg, which then closes itself off to any other sperm. Fertilization has occurred! Unless there are other eggs nearby to fertilize, as could be the case if fertility drugs are used, the unlucky extra sperm simply die off. Their part in the conception drama is, alas, over.

Remember that even under the best of circumstances, conception does not always occur!

Although there is now a fertilized egg, the conception process has a few more steps to it. First, the newly fertilized egg tumbles through the fallopian tube, ever dividing, until after a few days it enters the uterus. All this time, it is producing increasing amounts of hCG (human chorionic gonadotropin), a hormone that pregnancy tests measure for and that can be detected about two weeks later. After a few more days in the uterus, this ball of cells—now called a blastocyst—contains about a hundred cells and is ready to burrow into the uterine lining. If it successfully embeds itself, implantation has occurred, and it will grow here in the uterus for the next nine months.

If conception does not occur, the uterine lining will soon be shed (often with the tiny egg in it, called the corpus luteum) and you will menstruate. Then the whole cycle repeats itself all over again.

Can You Plan for a Boy or a Girl?

It seems that more lesbians hope for girl children than for boys. Unfortunately for us, it is the biological father's sperm that determines the sex of the child. The common wisdom is that alternative insemination produces more boys. This can seem true when using frozen sperm. One factor that may contribute to this is that most women inseminate only once or twice a cycle when using frozen sperm, as close to the time of ovulation as possible. Because the boy sperm, which carry the Y chromosome, are thought to swim faster but die faster, they have an advantage over the hardier, but slower-swimming girl sperm, which carry the X chromosome. Those boy sperm may be able to dart up there past their female counterparts and grab that waiting egg. If you are inseminating a few days before ovulation, particularly with fresh sperm, the girl sperm will have a better chance of hanging out and waiting for the egg, easily outliving the boy sperm.

RECOMMENDED READING

Beginning Life: The Marvelous Journey from Conception to Birth by Geraldine Lux Flanagan features incredible, highly magnified color pictures of the conception process.

The problem is that if you use the frozen goods, their shorter life span makes this kind of deliberation almost pointless. You really just have that window of a day or two of peak fertility to inseminate using frozen sperm, and you have to try it then, whatever your preference for the sex of the child. Fresh sperm, on the other hand, can live several days, even up to a week. So, theoretically, using fresh sperm—particularly over the course of the week leading up to ovulation—may increase your odds of having a girl.

In the end, this is all just speculation. In my own lesbian mom–baby group, of eight mothers, five had girls. Three of us used frozen sperm, one used fresh sperm from a known donor, and one had sex with a man. I had an IUI the morning after I ovulated and had a girl, which the odds would say was nearly impossible for a lesbian. When I meet women who have read my book and now have children, the number of boy children and girl children seems about equal. It did seem for a while that many more boy children were being born to lesbians, but I think in retrospect the imbalance might have been imagined. Certainly, there were more boy children being born within the dyke community than in the past—but there were lots more girls being born, too. In short, the gayby boom has produced lots more children of both sexes.

Are there ways to maximize your chances of having one sex or another? It's worth a try, if you feel really strongly about it. You could read books like *How to Choose the Sex of Your Baby*, but you'll find the methodology doesn't wholly apply to lesbian couples who aren't conceiving through heterosexual intercourse. Or you could spend many thousands of dollars having sperm "sorted" to weed out most of the female or male sperm in an ejaculate—if you can find a company willing to do this for a lesbian couple. It has a higher success rate for producing girl children than boy children. There are even kits available online from companies that promise to at least better your odds. One such option is available from www.genselect.com. But remember to read the small print and really understand that there are no guarantees for one sex or another. Until a sperm-sorting method is developed that is 100 percent guaranteed and affordable for the average woman, you'll have to accept the child the goddess sends your way! If you can't bear the thought of having a boy child, think about adopting a girl. Of course, once you give birth to a child of either sex, you will find you love it for who they are and who they will become. And since lesbians are such wonderful parents, you will have much to give a child of either sex. Lucky kids!

Checking Your Fertility

To any woman starting to try to get pregnant, I would say, read and learn about your own fertility. Once you really begin this process, you will be better able to advocate for yourself. —Joyce

Because as a lesbian you generally have only one or two tries each month to attempt to become pregnant, it is imperative that you learn how to tell if and when you're fertile. This is not hard to do, and soon you will become an expert at it.

There are several ways you can check to determine when you are most fertile. It will take a cycle or two to become familiar with them and decide which methods you will use as conception tools.

Cervical Mucus

Once I began tracking my fertile mucus, I realized just what this goo I had always noticed actually was! It was a great indicator of when I was about to ovulate. It was like, here comes the mucus, phone up the sperm bank! —Natalie

One of the most reliable fertility signs is cervical mucus. Even if you think you don't know a thing about it, you have probably been vaguely aware of its presence. Have you ever noticed white stains in your underwear, or gooey stuff appearing on the toilet paper you've used? What you've seen is cervical mucus, and you've probably just taken it in stride as a regular bodily function and not thought to question its varying appearance. But cervical mucus is one of the keys to conception. Therefore, it warrants closer inspection here.

If you have a partner, and you both want her to get involved, you can put her in charge of fertility checks and charts. She can be the one to read the pee sticks, check your cervical position, and analyze your mucus. She can be in charge of temperature-taking and maintaining your temperature chart. This will help her feel involved even though you're the one whose body this all depends on!

Cervical mucus is produced by all ovulating women. The quantity and consistency will vary from woman to woman, cycle to cycle, and day to day. Your mucus can be affected by the weather, or even by the stress of trying to conceive, so even within individual women, each cycle will be different. And some women never produce much, in which case this will not be the most useful fertility sign to track. Still, it is amazing how variations in the amount and consistency of your mucus can predict how you get pregnant.

Here are the phases that a typical woman's mucus goes through:

- During your period, you will not notice much mucus, because you are bleeding—but get ready for changes soon to come.

- In the days right after your period, you will find that you either have no mucus or are very dry at your vaginal opening. There probably won't be any "show" in your underpants on these days.
- After a few days, you may begin to get what is called "sticky" mucus. It can be rubbery looking, or kind of clumpy, but not very wet or gooey. You are not yet fertile.
- Next, your mucus may become creamy, looking somewhat like hand lotion. It may put a spot in your underwear. You are getting fertile at this point.
- Now you will probably be close to the midpoint of your cycle, ready for the appearance of fertile mucus. It will be very different from the creamy stuff of a few days before. It will probably be fairly clear (or have a slight yellow tinge), and it may have an elastic quality like the white part of a chicken egg. If you've never noticed what raw egg white looks like, crack open an egg and examine its consistency. Touch the egg white with your fingers and note its elasticity and translucence. This will help you know what to look for, albeit in much smaller quantities, when your next cycle rolls around. If you place some of your own fertile cervical mucus between your fingers it should stretch out at least an inch, if not several inches. You may notice it most the first thing in the morning, when you awaken. Or sometimes when you wipe yourself after urinating, you may see small globs of it on the toilet paper. This stretchy mucus is called *spinnbarkeit*; we will call it *spin* for short. It may sound odd at first, but soon you will be asking yourself, "Am I spinny yet?" Spin is one of the best indicators of fertility.

So What about Spin?

Why should you care about spin, and what does it do for you? If you were to look at different kinds of cervical fluid under a microscope, you would see that mucus acts very much like a barrier to sperm for most of your cycle. It's like a tangled web that sperm gets caught in. This is not fertile mucus.

When you get spin (or fertile mucus), it's as if the channel doors have opened. Suddenly, there are pathways for the sperm to swim through into your cervix on the way to meet the egg. It's as if our bodies have a defense mechanism for keeping sperm out until the egg is ready. Once your body lets you know, by producing spin, that ovulation is beckoning, your window of opportunity narrows. If you are in your twenties or early thirties, you may get spin for several days, but if you are older, you may notice it only for a day or so. Some women who are ordinarily a bit dehydrated (perhaps from drinking too much coffee and caffeinated soft drinks) may find that simply drinking more water helps them produce more mucus, especially in the hot summer months.

Can you make your body produce more spin? Start by eating well and drinking enough water. Then feel free to check out all the various folk remedies you'll hear about from friends and on the Internet. But use some common sense, ladies. While it may be a smart idea to think about acupuncture and specially pre-pared and brewed Chinese teas, drinking too much cough medicine to thin your mucus probably isn't so great for your health.

I would recommend beginning to learn about your mucus right after you finish a period. This will allow you to track a cycle from beginning to end.

After ovulation, your spin dries up quickly due to rising progesterone levels and decreasing estrogen levels. For the rest of the month, you will have somewhat dry or thick mucus, designed by your body to block entry to the cervix once again. And you are no longer fertile till after your next period.

Other Kinds of Mucus

Sometimes you hear reports about women who produce "hostile mucus," and for them it's even harder to conceive, as their mucus does not seem to want to allow sperm in at all. Or it may just kill the sperm on contact! While it may seem humorous that lesbians would produce sperm-killing mucus, for women trying to conceive it is maddening. You can only really find out if this is the case by taking a sample of your vaginal fluid right after an insemination and having it analyzed. If the sperm in the fluid are all dead, and they were alive before you inseminated, you know you've got a problem. Talk to your doctor about how best to remedy this.

VAGINAL INFECTIONS

If you have any strange- or bad-smelling discharge, or suspect you have a yeast or vaginal infection, get it checked out and cleared up at least a month before you try to conceive.

AROUSAL FLUID

The fluid your body produces when you're sexually excited is *not* the same as fertile mucus! Arousal fluid is produced by your body when you're turned on, and it acts as a lubricant during sex play, but it does not have the same qualities as fertile mucus, and it isn't known to provide channels for the sperm to swim through.

LUBRICANTS

If you are expecting to inseminate within a day or two, it's best to avoid heavy use of lube during sex play. According to Cathy Winks and Anne Semans, authors of *The Good Vibrations Guide to Sex*, the preservative ingredients in all lubes are capable of killing sperm—even in water-based lubes that do not contain nonoxynol-9. Of course you do not want to use any lubricant or lubricated condoms containing nonoxynol-9, which kills sperm. Even though nonoxynol-9 has been shown to increase rates of HIV transmission in some cases, it is still found in some brands of lubricated condoms. Check the fine print on all product containers and wrappers. The last thing you want to discover, on the day you're about to inseminate, is that you used a spermicide the night before!

Things That Might Affect Your Fertility

Some women have minor or even serious health problems that may curtail their ability to get pregnant. These include endometriosis, pelvic inflammatory disease, and fibroids. You should consult a doctor if you have previously suffered from any such conditions or if you have ever had surgery on any part of your reproductive tract. Before you jump on the conception roller coaster, it's good to know your chances of becoming pregnant, and how to maximize your odds.

However, there are a number of commonsense things that any woman can do to boost her everyday odds of getting pregnant. These include avoiding radiation, toxins (including those in paints), and overexposure to CRT computer monitors. You should also cut back on caffeine, alcohol, and marijuana, all of which have been proven to suppress fertility. Stop smoking cigarettes for all the reasons you already know—and for some new ones: It's detrimental to your fertility, and it will harm your unborn child. And get your partner to stop, too, since secondhand smoke is unhealthy for all. If you feel you just can't stop smoking, ask yourself if you want to smoke more than you want a baby. Parenting will constantly require that you put your baby's needs in front of your own. If you can't do that now by stopping smoking, you're already on the wrong path. (Am I lecturing you, ladies? You betcha.)

Douching is also a poor idea, since it changes the pH balance of your vagina, the last thing you want to be doing right now. Be healthy and fit, but don't overexercise or diet—don't shock your body just when you need its cooperation the most.

And stress? I found the stress of trying to conceive unbelievable, and it really whacked my body out. Since stress is certainly going to be part of your life during this process, it's best to find ways to minimize it wherever you can. Gentle massage? Meditation? Laughter? Yes, yes, yes! For more on stress relief, see chapter 5, Surviving the Roller Coaster: Ten Tips to Keep You Sane.

Taking Your Temperature

After you've been doing this for a while, you may wish for a morning where you can just bound out of bed without taking your temperature. Just check for a month every now and then so you don't burn out on it. —Ava

Taking your temperature every morning is like boot camp for fertility awareness. Exciting for one cycle, obsessive for a few more, then merely annoying, till you just want to throw the thermometer across the room. And your girlfriend may well do just that after being awakened every morning by that little beep-beep at 7:00 A.M. Instead of using an everyday thermometer, you'll need a special basal body thermometer, which measures tenths of degrees within the 95-to-99-degree range. These are available in most drugstores for under $25. I like the digital ones for their ease of use, though some clinics recommend only the mercury variety, which may be more accurate but are a little harder to read.

Before you ovulate, your temperature is low, but a surge of progesterone in your body after ovulation causes your temperature to shoot up quickly. If you get pregnant, your temperature will stay high (or rise even higher). If you do not, it will generally fall dramatically the day before or the day you actually bleed. Taking your temperature and noticing this drop lets you know your period is coming—which is, of course, quite upsetting when you're trying to get pregnant! Take your temperature first thing in the morning, before you move around at all, even to go to the bathroom. This is very important if you want accurate and consistent results. Charting your cycle a few times will bring you in tune with what these slight but important variations in temperature mean for you, and you will begin to notice a distinct pattern to your body's temperature. This is also a surefire way of determining if, indeed, you are even ovulating, which is a good thing to know before you start the rest of this process. If you don't notice a spike, you're probably not ovulating. If this is the case, you will need to start taking some type of fertility medication to remedy this.

How charting works: You will fill out a special chart that records your waking temperature. Each day you'll place a dot on the chart to record your temperature, taken at exactly the same time every day. Connect the dots and you will see the natural rhythm of your body over the course of a full menstrual cycle. Start each chart with your period. Note the dates of your spin and the date of your surge. Your chart will typically look something like the example provided here, though please remember that every woman's cycle length is different. You'll find a blank chart in the appendix; feel free to make copies. You can also find and print free copies of a nicely detailed fertility chart at www.thefertilityshop.com. Look for it in the site map; it is listed as Printable BBT Cycle Chart.

Try charting the different phases of mucus on your temperature chart, and you will begin to see how your fertility signs all work together!

I have to warn you that charting your periods can make you terribly obsessive. And also, if you're like me, the stress of trying to get pregnant may cause your cycles, and therefore your data, to veer all over the place. After about four tries, I didn't chart my periods anymore except to note when I had spin, and the days when I surged, when I inseminated, and when I bled. Other women find charting their cycles to be a comforting process. For the first month or two, I think it's a useful tool, but if the charts start annoying you, don't worry about completing them. Some sperm banks and clinics ask you to fill out one every month. But hey, it's your body and your money, so do what works for you. Also, please note that while ovulation kits (see below) have become the most popular way of determining the time of insemination, only by taking your temperature will you know if you have actually ovulated and released that all-important egg.

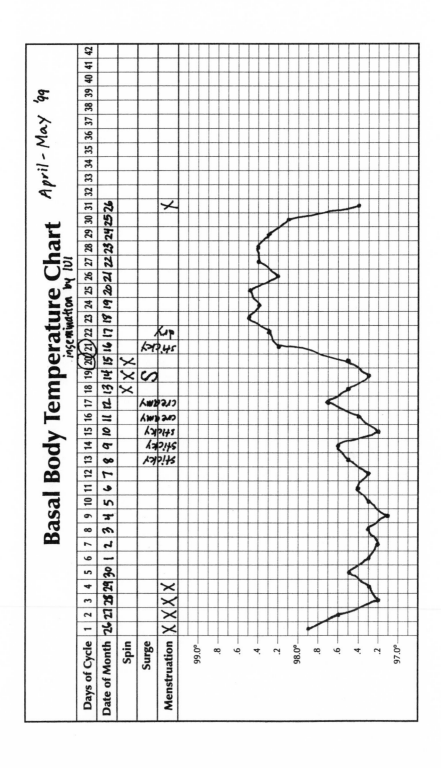

Ovulation Kits

One of the easiest and most convenient methods of testing for your ovulation is to use ovulation predictor kits, or OPKs. Some women call
them, less formally, "pee sticks." Several brands are available in most
large drugstores, though you may have to ask for them at the pharmacy
counter. HMO pharmacies also stock some brands. These kits are extensively available online, often from drugstore sites that explain in great
detail how to use them. The most basic kits cost $25–$40 for a month's
supply.

Most ovulation kits contain some variation of a test stick that measures the amount of LH, or luteinizing hormone, in your system. As LH is
in fact the catalyst for your body to ovulate, it appears in your urine most
strongly right before ovulation. The test sticks are plastic and usually
about five inches long. You pee onto an area on one side of the stick, and
a window on the other side displays the result after a few seconds.
Usually, you do the test around noon, after you have held your urine for
a few hours—this is to allow hormonal levels to build up in your pee. It's
not recommended that you use your first pee of the morning, since it often
won't indicate that you are surging, even if you are. Make sure you read
the instructions that come with each type of kit you buy, since they may
vary. And it's a good idea to test twice a day during your most fertile days.

The strong appearance of LH (or luteinizing hormone) in your urine
right before ovulation is called your surge. (The surge is discussed earlier
in this chapter.) When you show signs of a surge, you are about to ovulate within 12 to 24 hours. If you test and no line appears in the window,
either you are not about to ovulate or you have already ovulated. If a
faint line appears, ovulation is still a few days away; you should keep testing until the line is as dark as or darker than the test line. You are waiting
for the darkest blue line to appear before you take any action.

Note that it can take a month or two of using a particular product to
familiarize yourself with the shades produced by its test results, and even
these can vary by batch. If you are unsure about a test kit's accuracy, test
again a few hours later with a new stick. The darker the line appears, the
closer you are to ovulation. If the test line appears to be equally dark two
days in a row, you have probably caught the surge as it rises and falls. This
may be especially true if you test twice a day and see a surge at night and
again the following morning. I know some women who test only once a
day, to save money. If you are really experienced at this, know your body

well, and use the tests mainly as a backup, you can test once a day—but be aware that you may indeed miss signs of your surge.

My own inclination was always to inseminate as soon as the surge stick turned blue. I was so excited to see signs of my surge that I wanted to get busy making a baby immediately. I was forgetting that a surge only predicts your ovulation—it doesn't announce its arrival. It is more than a bit tricky to pinpoint the perfect time in each cycle until after it passes, so you may miss the moment in some months. Certainly, the more times you can inseminate in each cycle, the better your chances. It's easy to get into a tizzy trying to identify your optimum day for inseminations, especially when you are having intrauterines done at a clinic and can afford only one try a month. Some women try right at their peak, others wait a day, some even two, while still others like to inseminate a day before their surge, in part to better the odds of having a girl. What seems to work for another woman may not work for you.

Here is my own crazy conception story: For six months I inseminated after my surge and before my ovulation, and I had no luck. The time I actually got pregnant, I was convinced I'd waited too long, as it was a day or so after the peak of my surge, my cervix was partially closed, and I felt sure I had already ovulated. In fact, I remember sitting in the Castro Theatre in San Francisco, feeling midpain and thinking I should probably call the clinic and cancel my IUI scheduled for the next morning. I had little hope that the egg I felt popping would be able to live till the next morning. But I kept the appointment, and I got pregnant. Either I was extremely lucky or I had been inseminating too early on previous tries. Or perhaps I merely felt my follicles swelling and the egg hadn't actually released yet. Or, as I like to tell people, my daughter was born from an Amazon egg. In any case, relying just on the pee sticks to predict ovulation is not as effective as combining those results with other fertility signs.

Many women want to test two, or even three, times a day when they're sure they're about to surge. I know the temptation to go a little crazy and blow through a whole pack of these strips in a few days. And give yourself permission to do that, if you need to, sometimes. But do keep in mind that the stress of constantly monitoring your impending ovulation may actually delay it! And look for a pattern in your ovulation, if possible. For example, I have always tended to ovulate in the late afternoon or evening, and many women report a similar pattern. This can help you predict how much time you have from the first sign of your surge to the optimal insemination moment.

Whatever type of kit you try initially, don't be afraid to try a different one the next month. Different kits work better for different women. Some women find that the line measuring the surge never gets as dark as the dark-blue test line in some of the cheaper kits. Some women prefer to use a kit that contains four or five test strips, while others buy the one-day kit. You'll find that many online bulletin boards and online drugstore sites (such as the aforementioned www.thefertilityshop.com) publish product reviews. Two of the most popular brands of ovulation kits are Clearblue Easy and Ovu-Quick. I recommend Ovu-Quick, but both are favorites in the lesbian community. The Clearplan website, www.Clearplan.com, is handy for ordering their products and for reading basic fertility information.

Also available online are various models of fertility monitors, which cost about $200. You will need to buy special test strips for these monitors that are similar to the pee sticks mentioned above. The monitor produces a reading of where you are in your cycle, and whether it's your optimum time to inseminate. Women with especially long cycles will not be able to use these monitors.

There are also affordable devices (around $40) that measure the hormonal content of your saliva. Other devices let you test your cervical mucus. When you are surging, your dried saliva appears fernlike under a microscope, similar to the pattern that frost makes on a window. This *ferning* is a sign that you have fertile mucus—the kind that sperm will be able to swim through most easily. Testing your saliva as a fertility awareness tool is best done in conjunction with another method. In addition, there are fertility "watches"; a video based on the book *Taking Charge of Your Fertility*, by Toni Weschler; and various other contraptions, herbs, and books you can buy that supposedly improve your chances of conceiving.

Do you need any of these items? That's a decision only you can make, based on the size of your budget and your willingness to experiment. Will buying any of these items help you get pregnant faster? Maybe, if they help you understand how your body works, thus maximizing your chances of conception. If some of these things had been available when I was trying to get pregnant, you can bet I would have bought them. Compared to even a few years ago, there is a tremendous wealth of products and information available today.

Will you get pregnant if you use only the ovulation predictor kits? If you are ovulating, and you use the OPK correctly, and don't inseminate too soon (but as close to ovulation as possible), your odds are as good as if you use additional fertility tools.

Other Fertility Signs

There are additional fertility signs you can check for, but it is unnecessary to do so unless you're really a stickler for details. But, then, aren't most of us obsessive when we're trying to conceive? I certainly was. I became very familiar with my cervix when I was trying to get pregnant. (And I haven't checked it out since.) At the very least, you'll learn some interesting new facts about the female body.

Let's start with the degree of openness of your cervix. This will bear close inspection, particularly if you're using a speculum during your insemination. Normally, your cervix appears closed, but as you approach peak fertility it will gradually open, and you may see it covered with, or oozing, fertile mucus. If your cervix is really wide open, this is a good indication that you are fertile! On several insemination attempts I was delighted to hear that my cervix was wide open, and I sent those little sperm strong messages to go ahead and swim on up there.

Make sure you stock up on, or order, ovulation kits well in advance of when you may need them! The last thing you want is to miss a month because you ran out of kits.

Feel free to ask whoever is doing your insemination if they can see your cervix, and how it looks. If the same person does your inseminations on more than one occasion, they will become a helpmate to you in understanding this fertility sign. You can also examine the angle of your cervix, which sits higher and feels softer when you're fertile. This one stumped me, I'll admit.

Some women regularly feel their egg burst through the ovarian wall at the height of their fertility. This is called *mittelschmerz* (midpain), and you will most often feel it on just one side of your body, sometimes for as long as a few hours. I regularly feel this pain— it's almost as if someone is digging a finger into my side and twisting it around. No, it's not gas, or a side-stitch, it's midpain! And it's an amazing fertility sign. If you can do an insemination right around the time you feel this pain, especially if it is your cycle's second insemination, you should consider your timing right on track.

In addition, some women will feel increasingly sexual as their ovulation approaches. It's as if nature were letting you know that now is the time to try! Personally, I have never felt so lushly sexual in my life as when I began trying to get pregnant and knew ovulation was near. Even a few years after the birth of my daughter, when I get this midcycle sexual rush, I want to make another baby.

Other secondary fertility signs may include a bit of spotting, water retention, and breast tenderness. You may always have experienced a small degree of many of these signs but never noticed them or thought to associate them with anything in particular. But believe me, by the time you have tried to get pregnant at least a few times, you will know them all, and all too well!

RECOMMENDED READING

Taking Charge of Your Fertility, *by Toni Weschler. Although the book has a heterosexual focus and the author talks a lot about "when to have sex with your husband," her careful examination of every fertility sign, her lengthy explanation of fertile mucus—complete with pictures—and her reassuring tone make this book a good investment.*

4

Getting the Goods

I don't remember semen being yellow. But then I never poured it into a vial, froze it for ten months, then thawed it in a baggie. It's a strange thing this yellow liquid, the bodily fluid of a stranger. What was he thinking when he shot his wad? Is he somewhere now wondering about his sperm? Is he at this very moment wondering if a woman somewhere is inseminating with his seed? Well, we are! Here we are in Boston, and we are!
—*from* Buying Dad, *by Harlyn Aizley*

Sperm: The Necessary Ingredient

Sperm. It's a subject many of us have shied away from most of our lives. But now that you've made the decision to get pregnant, it's a necessity. How do you get it? How much will you pay for it? How do you ask a guy to give you some? What do you do with it once you have it? This chapter will explore how to obtain sperm, how to keep it viable so that it can work its magic, how much it'll cost you, and how to protect yourself legally in the process.

What Are Sperm?

Sperm (or more formally, spermatozoa), are continually produced by a man. Each day, a man can produce millions of them. Sperm are produced in the testes, which hang outside a man's body, and optimally do not touch one another or the body. Although sperm must be kept at body temperature once ejaculated, the normal human body temperature is too hot for their production. It takes at least ten days for sperm to be produced and to mature, and during this time they sit waiting in coiled tubes in an outer part of the testes called the epididymis. They are then believed to release tiny amounts of carbon dioxide to temporarily paralyze themselves until they're needed in an ejaculate. When this time comes, sperm are mixed with fluids from several glands including the prostate, which help them along their journey into the vagina. They are shot through the man's urethra during ejaculation, ready for their mission of fertilization in the female body. Within a single ejaculate, a significant percentage of sperm must be shaped normally (proper morphology), able to move forward quickly (motility and progression), and present in high enough numbers that a woman stands some chance of getting pregnant. A semen analysis and a sperm count will let you know these factors. For a small fee, most clinics or sperm banks can do these tests onsite with an appointment. You will not have to wait long for your results, usually just a few hours or one business day.

Sperm Are in the Semen

When a man ejaculates, the fluid he produces is called semen. Semen has a number of components, including sperm, sugars, salts, and other secretions. Every man produces different quantities of live and healthy sperm, which is measured as his sperm count. This can vary widely from day to day, but a typical ejaculate contains millions of sperm—often up to 200 million. However, only a small percent of this seemingly huge number may actually be viable. Often, large numbers may be misshapen, dead, or unable to travel in a forward direction up and toward your waiting egg.

What Is Semen?

Semen is the liquid ejaculate of an adult male. It is composed of sperm, of course, and the agents that carry it out of the body—including body fructose (a form of sugar), salts, white blood cells, and other secretions of the prostrate gland and seminal vesicles. Semen is an alkaline body fluid, with a normal pH balance in the range of 7.2–8.0. Semen is also measured for viscosity, the rate at which it liquefies. The thicker, or more viscous, a man's semen, the more difficult it will be for sperm to travel in it. Therefore, especially for insemination purposes, you will want to make sure the viscosity of your donor's semen allows the sperm to travel easily through it. Its liquefaction should be complete within 10–30 minutes of ejaculation.

When you use freshly ejaculated semen, or a vial of the "unwashed" frozen stuff from the sperm bank, you are inseminating with sperm still in the semen. However, if your midwife "spins" sperm from your donor, or you buy "washed" sperm from a bank—often specifically for a procedure such as an intrauterine insemination, where the sperm are fed more directly into the uterus—the mix will be different. In these cases, you are being inseminated with a high-density mixture of sperm, often in an egg-yolk cryopreservation mixture. This is because the midwife or clinic has spun out of the semen the slower-swimming sperm and any that may be nonviable. In this book, I'll talk primarily about sperm, as opposed to semen, since it is the sperm that actually causes you to get pregnant.

Known Versus Unknown Donor: The Big Decision

One of the biggest decisions you will make in trying to get pregnant is whether to use a known or an unknown donor. This should be a decision on which you spend some time. Don't rush into the first available option just because you want to get started. How you create your child will have long-lasting implications for your life, so it's best to consider all the issues involved. You should take special care to thoroughly examine the legal implications if you use a known donor.

Using a Known Donor

There are many reasons why women may choose to use a known donor:

- You know how the donor looks and acts
- You are likely to be able to try inseminating more than once during a cycle, bettering your chances of conception
- Fresh sperm are more active, so you may conceive sooner
- Your child can have a relationship with the donor as he or she grows up, if both parties want this
- You have a male friend who really wants to help out or be involved
- You can use a gay man as your donor, whereas most sperm banks use only heterosexual men
- The nonbiological mom may feel more in control of the process if she picks a friend of hers as the donor
- The donor may be genetically linked to the nonbiological mother in a female couple (he could be her brother, perhaps), thereby guaranteeing her some biological connection to the child
- You cannot afford to buy frozen sperm or use the services of a clinic
- You feel you have no access to a sperm bank or clinic that meets your needs

Of course, you may think you have the perfect male specimen in mind, but when you ask him to donate, he says no. Or he might inform you that he has HIV or some other disease. Or he might initially agree, then back out. You will have to see how it goes—and don't be devastated if the perfect donor doesn't work out. Whoever your donor ends up being, your baby will still be the perfect baby for you.

It's important to remember that different women, all having different experiences, have vastly varying opinions on whether you should use a known or unknown donor. This is a decision only you and your partner can make. If you put ten lesbian moms in a room, they will tell you ten ways they came to their own decision about this particularly important path to parenthood.

I initially wanted to use a known donor, but I changed my mind after three separate men had to come out to me as HIV-positive when I asked them. One even said he'd considered lying to me about his status because he wanted a child so badly. That scared me enough to only consider using a sperm bank from then on.

—Theresa

We had a close friend who took an AIDS test. He came over three days in a row and did his donation in a sterile dish. We did not consult any doctors, nor did we use any drugs. The donor sees our son every so often but does not want to be a significant part of his life. He knew right from the beginning that it was "right" to donate to us. —Patrice

Collecting Fresh Donor Sperm

The most usual scenario for donating fresh sperm is for the donor to come over, masturbate in the bathroom, and ejaculate into a container. Then he usually hands over the container and leaves, letting the woman or women get on with the insemination. Other men prefer to do their business at home, have one of the women drive over and pick it up, and take it back to her partner. Other men will personally deliver it, even on a motorcycle, with a sealed jar tucked inside their coat. Will sperm live through experiences like this? Yes, but you need to be careful.

Sperm should be collected from the donor in a smallish cup or bowl that is clean, at room temperature, and made of glass or plastic. No metal containers should be used. Make sure there is no soap or water present in the container. If it is to be transported, the container should be sealed and kept upright, so part of its precious content doesn't get spread out and wasted on the sides of the jar. Do not let it sit in direct sunlight. And make sure your donor does not use any lubricant while masturbating, as this can kill the sperm.

The collected sperm should be kept at body temperature until used. When transporting, the receptacle containing the sperm should be kept as close to a human body as possible to keep it warm. Fresh sperm can live up to a few hours once ejaculated, but it is best to use it immediately, or at least within an hour. To the lesbian eye, the quantity of semen in a single ejaculate may look rather small. As long as there is enough to fill a needleless syringe, you have more than enough to try to get pregnant! If your donor produces a larger quantity of ejaculate, make sure you use it all.

Asking a Guy to Be Your Donor

Initially, most women think it might be easier to just find a known donor to help them get pregnant. It seems more convenient, and certainly cheaper than buying sperm. Sometimes the right man will be in your life before you even decide to get pregnant. You'll ask him, he'll say yes, you'll inseminate, and then you'll get pregnant. That sounds so easy, and for some women it is. Typically, however, the experience can entail scouting around for a while. After thinking about what you are looking for in a donor, you will have to decide if anyone you know fits the bill. If they don't, you will have to continue looking.

How do you find a donor? My baby-crazed friend Andrea once stopped a guy at a crosswalk and asked him. He was cute and she liked his look. That might be a little extreme, but it's not entirely off base. It just proves a potential good donor can be found almost anywhere. He could be your partner's gay cousin, or a dear old straight friend who's already married with children. He could even be the guy who serves you your morning chai, so reliably at work on the very days you seem to be ovulating. The trick is to find someone whose health is good, who will actually work with you on this (because it will be work for him too), who will easily share a similar vision of his role in the life of your child, and whom you can talk with and trust. Realistically, he should be someone you or your partner have known for a while, as opposed to a random encounter. You'll want to know something about his health history, and how he conducts his life. To better protect yourself legally, it's best not to be reckless about who you ask.

Unfortunately, finding the right guy can take a while, especially if you and your partner disagree on whom to ask. And if you try to rush things with a man, the fit may not be good, and it won't work out for anyone involved. You might also wish to stay away from people in power relationships with you or your partner, such as a boss or important client.

If you feel that you aren't finding the right person, take a breather. You might need to take a wider look around at your circle of friends and acquaintances, or do a little self-promotion. Ask your friends if they know any great guys who might be interested. Make sure people know that you are looking and that you're ready to start. Be clear about what donating means to you, and what you expect from a donor.

When you do approach a man about being a donor, don't ask questions like "Have you always wanted to be a father?" This may give the wrong impression about the role you actually expect him to play. You might start by saying, "You know, I've been" (or "we've been") "giving a lot of thought to having a baby. I'm looking for a man to donate his sperm to me to help me get pregnant. Is that something you'd be interested in?"

Keep things light during the first conversation. Make sure you're clear that this is not about sex and that you're only looking for a sperm donation. Tell him a bit about what sperm donation entails—that it will mean health checkups for him, a sperm count, and legal forms to sign. It will mean he must put certain behaviors on hold, such as smoking pot and hot-tubbing, and he will be on call to make several deposits on your fertile days. Make sure he understands that he will not be considered the father (if this is in fact your intention), and that he has to be okay with that, now and forever. If he expresses interest, suggest that he think about it for a week and you will discuss it in more detail then.

Most responsible guys will want to ponder what this would mean to them before they commit. That's a good thing. You haven't made your decision lightly to ask him, so you'll want him to respond in kind. If he says yes right away, suggest he take a week to think things through any-way. Often, men who say yes too quickly back out later in the process when they see how much work they actually have to do, and you'll be even more disappointed in having to start all over again.

When you meet again, if he says yes, proceed with caution through the next phase of negotiations. If he says no, move on. There is no point in trying to cajole someone into changing his mind, as this could cause problems later. If he still says maybe, agree on when you can expect to have a firm answer; if he doesn't give you an answer by then, move on. Some guys will keep you hanging for a while if you let them. I let one male friend of mine keep me waiting half a year while he debated rather passively about his decision. He was my ideal candidate and remains to this day one of my favorite men. He really wanted children and was excited to proceed with me, but he didn't feel ready. Unfortunately, I wasted six precious reproductive cycles waiting for him. Almost ten years later, he still loves and wants children, but hasn't gotten around to it. Men have the luxury of fathering children into their later years. We women don't have the same ability. Stay in control of the process, and be assertive in making it happen for yourself. Be smart—treat a long-delayed response as a no and look for someone else to ask. Or use a sperm bank.

If your first choice for a donor says no right away, thank him for his honesty, and move on with no hard feelings. Don't even think of trying to get him to change his mind. Would you want someone trying to change your mind about having a child? I didn't think so.

Things to Think About When Using a Known Donor

YOU MUST SCREEN THE DONOR'S HEALTH YOURSELF

The onus is on you, for your health and the health of your baby, to make sure the donor is healthy. Many men agree to be a donor but balk at taking a battery of medical tests (which you will likely have to pay for if he's uninsured). You should screen your donor for the same conditions screened by any quality sperm bank: HIV, syphilis, hepatitis B and C, HTLV 1, cytomegalovirus (CMV), gonorrhea, chlamydia, mycoureaplasma, complete blood count, liver and kidney function, past medical history, family medical history, and blood type. Some sperm banks will perform semen analysis in their labs, often using guidelines established by the World Health Organization to evaluate fertility. Factors include the volume of semen ejaculated (at least 2 cc), its pH (7.2–8.0 is normal), and the morphology (size and shape) of the sperm. Sperm must be able to travel forward (referred to as progression), or they will never be able to swim upward to find the egg. On a scale of 1 to 3+, zero means there is no movement, 1 indicates the sperm are moving but not forward, 2+ equates to a slow forward motion, and by the time you reach 3+, the sperm are moving straight forward at a good clip. If you use a sperm bank, all these factors will already have been considered and measured, though you may have to ask to get such specific information. If you use a known donor, you're on your own. I know women who tried with a donor for a year or more before anyone considered getting his fertility tested, only to be told that his sperm were all abnormally shaped, had no progression, or were simply and sadly, dead.

YOU WILL HAVE TO TRUST HIS BEHAVIOR

This includes trusting that over the time you spend trying to get pregnant (whether that be a month or three years), he will engage only in safer-sex activities, curtail his consumption of drugs and alcohol, wear loose underwear, and avoid hot tubs to keep his sperm count up. Caffeine may actually improve sperm motility, as may certain vitamins. However, antibiotics and herbal supplements like Echinacea can reduce sperm counts. You may also wish to ask your donor to avoid either solo or partnered sex for a day or two before he ejaculates for your use. This will significantly help build up his sperm count. Between two and five days of abstinence is considered optimal. More than five days, however, may actually lower his sperm count.

Will you be comfortable talking with your donor about these basic issues, and especially his sexual practices? You need to be able to talk to him, and trust him, about these issues. If you tell him you want him to engage in safe sex while he is serving as a donor, you will need to negotiate what you mean by this. Some men define it as using a condom for anal intercourse—but may engage in other sex play without a latex barrier. Some practices that are effective in preventing HIV are not as effective in preventing other STIs, such as herpes. If he has a partner he is sexually active with, make sure that his partner, whether a man or a woman, is also following these guidelines.

You can find information on safer-sex practices for men from your local AIDS service organization, or online.

HE MAY NOT BE AVAILABLE WHEN YOU ARE OVULATING

Let's face it—people lead busy lives. Even men who give this a great deal of thought may find that they do not want to be on call for your purposes 24/7. If they have to travel for business, or are impulsive in recreational travel, you may find you are missing chances to inseminate. This can become extremely frustrating. A man may have a hard time understanding the tight timeline you need him to be on. It's best to spell this out very clearly beforehand. If you are vague about the commitment, he won't understand why you start freaking out if he doesn't return a phone call as soon as your ovulation predictor kit says "Go."

If you decide to use a donor who lives in another city, this may create big hassles for all involved. The logistics can be burdensome, with transportation and work schedules to plan around every month. Can your budget support this? Can your sanity? Can your timeline? I have known women who made it work, but it's a lot of effort. Some women prefer a long-distance donor. They may want a known donor but don't want him living too close by, especially in case he tries to eclipse the role of the nonbiological mother as the other parent. Bear in mind, when using a long-distance donor, that traveling may cause your ovulation time to shift. Those expensive plane tickets may prove useless if you ovulate the day before you're supposed to travel, or too many days after you return home from seeing the donor.

Kate Kendell Advises on Known Donors

Kate Kendell, Director of the National Center for Lesbian Rights, urges women to exercise much forethought in deciding whether to use an anonymous or a known donor. Both options have long-term implications for the kind of family you create. "Don't make an impulsive decision," she warns. When selecting a known donor, she says, "Don't pick a donor like you'd choose a roommate. All of us know this is no way to start a family." Kendell is clear that women about to start the insemination process should talk to other women who have been on this journey, particularly in their own geographic area. "I strongly urge a couple considering having children to canvas their social group as to how they made their choices, and why," she told me in an interview. She also tells women to be very clear in their conversations with potential known donors. Spend time together, she urges, and make sure you agree on basic childrearing philosophies—everything from whether your elementary school–aged son can wear nail polish to whether he will be circumcised as an infant. If you can't agree on issues like these, you should probably make the decision to look elsewhere for a donor or father. "Don't take a chance that things will just work out," she urges. The process of resolving differences in advance with a known donor can make all the difference later if conflicts arise. It's also extremely important, she says, that a known donor agreement be used. Although such documents may not be upheld in court, they are "enormously important," Kendell says, in "fleshing out the expectations and intentions" of the people involved. All lesbians considering using a known donor should consult with a knowledgeable attorney in their state. And don't trust that a known donor won't develop paternal feelings for a child later on—this can and does happen. Without documents to back up your intentions, the courts may award a known donor parental status.

> *My advice is to use a sperm bank rather than a known donor. Your donor, although he may sign away his rights, could come back and sue for paternity. A judge could reverse any agreement and reinstate his parental rights, granting him visitation and possibly joint custody. Don't doubt that this could happen to you. This is exactly what happened to us. It is not necessarily cheaper to use a known donor as opposed to a sperm bank. If a court case were to ensue it could run into thousands of dollars.*
>
> *—Wren*

Using a Known Donor Can Work Just Fine

Now that I've scared you, let me also add that most known donor arrangements work out just fine. Kendell says that the NCLR is seeing a decreasing number of lawsuits involving disputes with known donors. She thinks this is due to a "maturity of the process." A greater understanding of the risks and complications that can arise has caused people to be more mindful of the choices they're making, she says. For couples who know the donor well and have discussed every possible aspect of conflict in advance, it can be a rewarding experience for everyone involved. Women I know have had good experiences using a known donor. A good friend of mine just got pregnant with baby number two from her donor, and the donor is a valued addition to their family. Other women use brothers, uncles, or cousins of their partners, with nary a legal complication. Preparation and trust are essential, and sometimes taking a chance seems to be the only way you'll get your baby. It can also be a more humane and even humorous way to conceive than the sterile methods employed at a clinic:

> In the first month I tried to get pregnant I ovulated early. I called my donor to see if he could make an impromptu donation. Our donor was at work, but he took a break and came up with the goods, which were then promptly delivered to our house by his partner. My girlfriend took one look at the specimen and asked, "Is that all there is?" and our donor's partner got a little defensive, saying, "Well, he was a little stressed!" The things committed donors go through! —Jackie

> The first time we inseminated, we used a known donor and went to his house. My training as a counselor helped me listen both to the donor and to my partner as they expressed their feelings about their fears and apprehension over the unusual circumstances of what we were doing. I talked to the donor about the gift he was giving us and told him we could never forget this. But I had been with very few men before coming out, and the minute I looked into the cup that held his semen, I felt nauseated. The more nauseated I became, the more inept I became at managing the whole process. The turkey baster we had was entirely too big. I could not draw any sperm up into it but was only able to blow

bubbles into the semen. I finally swallowed hard, put some on my finger...and literally took the plunge. The next day, we bought a syringe, and the rest of our inseminations went great! —Angela

I'm white and my partner is Japanese American. When we decided that I would get pregnant, we asked her cousin to be our donor. That way we'd have a biracial child, and she could be related to the baby, too. We had legal papers drawn up but have never needed them. The donor, who lives in another city, acts as an "uncle" and sees our daughter a few times a year. It's been wonderful for all of us to see her grow up. —Hettie

When my son was four weeks old, his father took him two days a week for about three hours at a time. At nineteen months my son spent the night for the first time at his father's house. Most recently, his father spends two nights a week at our house, since he now lives a few hours away. All in all, it's an arrangement that's worked well for us. —Lara

A knowledgeable attorney in your own state or province can help you draw up documents for known donor and coparenting situations. Like any legal document, it should be especially tailored to your own personal situation.

The Father Factor

I met him through a support group for prospective gay and lesbian parents. We only knew each other for four months before we decided we'd like to coparent a child. We spent a lot of time together talking about all the issues involved and worked out a parenting agreement, which we have never had to refer to. I got pregnant the second time we tried. Our daughter splits the time between his house and mine. We have been extremely lucky that we get along so well, and we always tell people that we don't recommend doing things as quickly as we did! —Maddie

There is another choice besides using the services of a sperm bank or a donor friend to get pregnant. Certainly it is not an option that legal experts would consider sound; yet, for many women, it makes the most sense. This is to allow the man with whom you become pregnant to be involved as a father in your child's life.

While the lesbian party line tends to favor the fatherless route, and there is much more support today for women using anonymous donors, many women find the idea of raising a child without a father less than desirable. Some lesbians and bisexual women really want the involvement of a father in their children's lives. They may also want the financial and emotional support that men can bring to the equation, as well as the opportunity to share parenting responsibilities. Some single women may prefer to coparent with a man, or men, rather than wait for the perfect female companion to come along. And some lesbian couples may have as longtime friends a gay male couple with whom coparenting seems the natural choice for creating an extended family of parents to shower a child with love.

Just as there are many of us who seek a lesbian family relationship similar in structure to the stereotypical nuclear family, there are also many who are looking for ways to create a new family dynamic.

This might take the form of a family with two moms and two gay dads; a lesbian and a gay man coparenting together; a single lesbian parenting with a gay male couple; a straight woman coparenting with a gay man; or a lesbian or bisexual woman coparenting with a straight man. The woman who is the biological parent may receive the sperm in donation form or may actually have sex with the man who will be the biological father. The father may or may not be listed on the birth certificate, depending on the wishes of those involved.

Indeed, many men, both straight and gay, are looking for a way to father without having to parent full-time. Some may be actively searching for a woman with whom to share parenting through a prospective gay parents group. Check your local gay/lesbian magazines for such a group, look for listings on the Internet, or even start your own group. Other men may not even consider parenting an option until they are approached by a woman friend or a couple. Then, the idea may take hold and they grow to become wonderful, involved fathers forever thankful for this opportunity.

In fact, Kate Kendell of the NCLR says she is noticing a growing number of lesbian couples partnering in their parenting with gay male couples. One man is the biological father, and his partner is the other dad. One woman is the biological mother, and her female partner the co-mother. "The donor is considered the father from the beginning in these situations," Kendell says. How do people make such complex families work? "Parenting is a complex and sometimes difficult map to navigate," she reminds us, "especially if your parenting perspective needs to be modified by compromise with others." In these situations, she urges very honest and frank conversations with all parties right from the start, as well as proper legal documentation. It can be hard to know all the "what if's" in advance, but just creating a coparenting agreement can lessen potential conflicts later.

Using a Sperm Bank

If you've decided you want to use a sperm bank, where do you begin to find one? More banks are opening in the United States and Canada all the time. In other parts of the world you will have a harder time finding a sperm bank. And even if you do, there may be no way they will inseminate a "single" woman. However, many U.S. sperm banks ship internationally now, depending on the receiving country's regulations. If you live outside the U.S., contact a sperm bank and ask for their current policies and international protocols for shipping sperm. Canadians can use either Canadian or American sperm banks, but the rules about inseminating may be different in the two countries.

If you're in Europe, there are closer options, such as the Danish Cryos International Sperm Bank, which claims to be responsible for more than 10,000 births in over 40 countries since 1991. Be aware that some states in the U.S. may have laws that prohibit sperm banks from sending deliveries to any place other than a doctor's office. And those doctors may not be allowed to hand over the sperm to let you do home inseminations, or may require paperwork from the sperm banks that states it is okay for them to do so. It's really ridiculous that there are such restrictive policies about sperm, but we can hope that these laws will change soon.

Legally and healthwise, you are most protected by using sperm from a sperm bank. Not only is the donor tested repeatedly for diseases like HIV, but you can also be assured that his sperm health and mobility is good; and in many cases he has already produced other live children. It is also reassuring to know that the donor can never come after you for custody, since he has legally signed his rights away.

Of the sperm banks in North America, some are geared more toward straight couples experiencing fertility issues, while others were founded expressly for single women and lesbians. Most no longer care who their clients are. Word of mouth is probably the best way to decide which bank you'll be most comfortable using. After all, if friends of yours were treated well, you probably will be too. If you don't know any women using sperm banks, my recommendation is to contact some of the banks in this book's resources section, or to thoroughly peruse their websites and see what appeals to you. The amount of information online about sperm banks now is almost overwhelming. For good basic information, start with the informative website of the Sperm Bank of California, one of the country's oldest, and a bank started specifically by women to help other women conceive. Originally an offshoot of the Oakland Feminist Women's Health Center, it launched the first identity-release program in 1983. Find it at www.thespermbankofca.org.

Some women simply decide to use the nearest sperm bank, to avoid expensive shipping costs and the logistics involved with receiving and returning liquid-nitrogen tanks. My award for most convenient method of shipping goes to the Midwest Sperm Bank, which uses a courier service to deliver sperm to its clients in the Chicago area—free of charge! Now that's service!

For a list of recommended sperm banks, check the resources chapter.

Behind the Scenes at a Sperm Bank

When I was using a sperm bank to try to conceive, I always wondered what was happening beyond the front desk. I know my readers are also curious about how a sperm bank operates. Where and how is the sperm stored? Where do men go to make their deposits? I asked Cathy Winks, the Lead Health Worker at the Sperm Bank of California, to take me on a rare behind-the-scenes tour of its facilities.

Cathy meets me at the reception area, the large front desk where female clients generally buy their sperm or check in. Next we walk into one of the clinic's meeting rooms, and Winks gives me an overview of the clinic, its history, and its philosophy. The bank was founded in 1982 and is the only nonprofit sperm bank in the U.S. They pioneered the first identity-release program in the world, which allows children conceived by donor insemination to learn their donor's identity when they reach age 18. About half of the women using this sperm bank are lesbians, and about twenty percent are single moms. There are 20–25 active donors at any given time, managed by a donor coordinator. Winks says the bank finds donors by advertising in college papers and through online sites. Donors must undergo "rigorous and continual health testing," Winks emphasizes, and must make a year's commitment to the process. In addition, they must be over 5'6", since clinics have found that women are prejudiced against short donors and won't pick them! Only about ten percent of interested donors survive the rigorous screening process. "It's not a quick buck," Winks says with a smile.

Although a high percentage of clients live in California, the bank ships "anywhere we can legally clear customs," Winks says. Sperm stay viable in a liquid-nitrogen shipping tank for up to ten days—more than enough time to travel internationally and to be viable when needed, if ordered on a realistic timeline.

Most of the sperm at the bank is kept in a special tank room, in large color-coded floor tanks. The sperm in each tank are further classified by letters and names, as well as by date of deposit. It's all highly organized, and a bit surreal. To stand before these large tanks full of vials of frozen sperm is to feel, unavoidably, the potential for human life within. Hundreds of babies could be born from these vials. It is a rare moment, bearing witness to the dreams of so many lesbians, and I send a message of goodwill to the tanks full of frozen little swimmers. May they reach the women who need them, I hope, and bring dreams of babies to life. Cathy then opens one of the tanks and shows me how a metal cane is used to retrieve the small vials of sperm stored inside. These vials can be stored for about 50 years with no loss of viability. Liquid nitrogen wafts from the tank, and I peer inside at the many deposits. From these humble vials of sperm and the eggs inside our lesbian bodies grow our longed-for children. It's truly miracle making in the works.

Nearby sit large storage tanks of liquid nitrogen that are replenished every few weeks for the clinic's use. Smaller shipping tanks that weigh about 20 pounds and have traveled the world in the name of babymaking sit at the ready. A separate area, as law dictates, is reserved for sperm that is still under quarantine.

Next, we go into a room where new deposits are processed before they can be placed in liquid nitrogen. To freeze the sperm too quickly, a technician tells me, would "shock the sperm," so they prefer to "put it to sleep gently." The sperm are mixed with a freezing medium for cry-opreservation containing glycerol (which acts as an antifreeze), test yolk buffer (a combination of buffered salts and chicken egg yolk, which provides a good protective environment for the sperm), and antibiotic. I also get to see the room, currently empty, where men do the business of ejaculation. It's startlingly simple, with a small bed, a "deposit cup" at the ready, and a display of pornography, including *Victoria's Secret* and *Penthouse*, as well as *Freshmen* for the gay men. A privacy system prevents the men from being seen by women using the clinic's services. Fully 30 percent of the sperm stored at the bank is for client depositors, who will use their own sperm at a later date. It must first be quarantined for at least 180 days. These vials are kept separately from the general tanks of donated sperm.

The main office, with a few friendly workers and baby pictures adorning the walls, completes the tour. There are no frills here, just a committed staff and sperm at the ready. Because inseminations are no longer performed at this bank, much of the Sperm Bank of California's business comes from online orders. Reflecting this, its website is very savvy, and includes a hefty amount of information on fertility awareness. A doctor's signature is required by all of this bank's clients to ensure that women are in good health prior to beginning insemination. Winks reminds me that, for a slightly older woman, good general health is no guarantee of the health of her eggs. After all, these eggs have been with her since before she was born, and they significantly decline in quality starting at age 40. For many women, she says gently, "This can be a harsh reality."

Winks has some final words of wisdom for women contemplating this route to conception. Be realistic, she says, of what your expectations are, and how long it could take to become pregnant. "Even young fertile (straight) couples having well-timed intercourse have at most a 25 percent chance of getting pregnant each time," Winks says. "A lot of ducks have to be in a row for a woman to get pregnant." As I did, Winks urges women to try at home for a few times to become familiar with the experience, and then step up their odds by trying an intrauterine at a clinic. "Take measured steps to optimize your situation," she urges. After all, the sperm bank can only do so much to help you along your journey. The rest is up to you—and the sometimes elusive, always magical wonders of fertilization.

Words of Advice from Maura Riordan,
Past Director of the Sperm Bank of California

Preparing for insemination can be very stressful. It's critical that women find the sperm bank that feels like the "right fit" for their needs. The importance of feeling a sense of control over the process and knowing that the sperm bank you're using is not just a business, but a supportive environment, cannot be underestimated. Fortunately, times are changing, and the sperm-banking industry is much less homophobic than it once was, but there are still a number of banks that aren't accustomed to working with lesbians and may use language (and make assumptions) based on heterosexual bias. It's important to shop around for the right sperm bank, which includes being open to the possibility of working with a bank in another state. Currently, sperm banks in urban areas such as San Francisco, Boston, and New York are most likely to work regularly with single women and lesbian couples and are better equipped to make the experience a positive and supportive one. The bottom line is that lesbians can and should expect to be treated respectfully and welcomed warmly by whatever bank they use.

Questions to Ask of a Sperm Bank

There are several basic questions you will need answered before you decide on a sperm bank:

HOW OUT CAN YOU BE?

If the sperm bank assumes its clientele is straight, you may have to do some educating, especially if you have an involved partner who comes to all your appointments. You may just be the bank's or clinic's first out lesbian couple, and they'll adjust accordingly. With the gayby boom raging on, you certainly won't be their last! However, if the bank or clinic is just downright hostile to the idea of inseminating lesbians, look elsewhere. With the ability to have sperm shipped from several lesbian-friendly banks across the United States directly to your living room, there's no reason to face homophobia where you don't have to. See chapter 13, Resources, for the best lesbian-friendly sperm banks.

HOW MANY DONORS DO YOU HAVE?
HOW MANY ARE ACTUALLY AVAILABLE?

These are two different questions, and the difference is important. One sperm bank I tried had 20 to 25 active donors on record, but many of the more desirable donors were simply not available for use. Most of these were donors who were willing to be known when the child turned 18, and they were in high demand. Women had already reserved their sperm for months in advance. You simply were unable to order their sperm, even though they were still listed as available. Luckily, these days, most banks frequently update their donor lists on their websites, and they note when a donor's quantity is low. If you see a donor listed as "limited quantity," pick a different donor. You may face huge disappointment if you've decided on a dream donor, and two months of trying later, his supply has run out.

> The policy of one bank we used was to encourage women to pre-pay for sperm, sometimes for up to six months ahead of time. This effectively put several highly desirable donors out of circulation. This was a terribly frustrating revelation for me, as I had spent days deliberating over donor choices, only to find my top picks were all unavailable. I had to really change my expectation for what kind of donor I was willing to use. Sometimes during the stress of the moment you are willing to compromise, but when I realized I was using a donor whose ethnicity and family health history were not what I really wanted, I had to step back and rethink my decision. Soon afterward, I changed sperm banks entirely and got my top donor pick. Three months later, I was pregnant. —Gerri

ARE YOUR DONORS WILLING TO BE KNOWN?
IF SO, AT WHAT AGE CAN THE CHILD KNOW?

There are certainly many more donor choices available to you if you *don't* ever want to know your donor's identity. That is because it is a relatively new idea to let children eventually meet their donor fathers.

Typically, many donors have been college students just looking to make a little extra money and then walk away. As more and more women use sperm banks, however, the common wisdom of using only unknown donors has changed. Many more mothers would like their children to have the option of meeting their donor one day. There are still few men willing to consider the possibility that eventually grown-up offspring may come knocking on their door. Increasingly, however, women are choosing donors who are willing to be known—sometimes called "yes" donors—if only to give their children the option of finding the men who have contributed to their existence.

The standard age at which a child can meet a "yes" donor father is 18. In rare situations, the child can meet the donor sooner. Rainbow Flag Health Services in California gives you the donor's contact information when your baby is just a few months old.

As a personal note, I'd like to add that in our haste to create families, I feel many lesbians are willing to deny their children the opportunity to seek their biological roots. Knowing many adoptees who as adults were almost frantic to find their biological parents has taught me the wisdom of not imposing our own limitations on our children. The fact that we create these children and want them to grow up in a lesbian family does not remove their need to know their origins—whether or not we approve. Some lesbian couples prefer to use "no" donors so the nonbiological mother can feel secure that no other parent lurks on the horizon. Do whatever is right for your family. But know that early studies show that most couples are very happy with their choice to use a "yes" donor—and almost every single mom is. Nonbiological moms feel the most hesitation about having their child meet their donor, but regrets are generally few. ("Choosing Identity-Release Sperm Donors: The Parent's Perspective 13–18 Years Later," by Scheib, Riordan, and Rubin.) If we use donors who are willing to be known, our children can grow up secure in the knowledge that, should they choose to seek their donor fathers, they will be able to do so one day.

Donor Information

Here is an example of an unknown donor's information. As you can see, what you will know about half of your child's genetic makeup is initially quite small:

Donor # 2213
Race/Ethnicity: Caucasian/German/English
Hair Color/Texture: Light Brown/Wavy
Eye Color: Blue
Skin Tone: Fair
Blood Type: A+
Height: 6'1"
Weight: 185 lbs
Occupation: Fireman
Interests: Nature, Swimming, Film

Some banks also offer a small amount of commentary on the donor's parents' health, as well as his personality and physique, by using terms like "long-limbed," "outgoing," and "witty."

For known donors, you may find the initial information listed will be about the same, but once you narrow down your choices, the bank will provide a more detailed family health history for you. Often this will also contain several pages of information, which may include the donor's favorite foods and colors, as well as his reasons for becoming a donor. If you can read these forms at the clinic, there is generally no fee, but if you want a photocopy, most banks charge up to $20 each for a printout of only several pages. More information may be available on many bank's Web pages. Some, such as the Midwest Sperm Bank, do not charge for either a short profile or the longer medical/genetic profile. They also offer a free, photo-assisted donor selection that helps you imagine what your features will look like blended with his. Pacific Reproductive Services (PRS) offers a longer donor form for $15. They also offer, for $30 each, and for their anonymous donors only, audio CDs of individual donors speaking for 15 minutes about their family history, why they decided to become a donor, and other facts you might find interesting. A photo of the donor as a child costs $35. Not to be outdone, California Cryobank, which has a very large number of donors, updates its website listings every few hours, lists whether the donor has produced other pregnancies, and marks its brand-new donors with a red star. You can also request a report of the donor's facial features and download an audio file of the donor speaking. It's truly amazing how technology has empowered women in the sperm-buying and clinic-choosing process. But, alas, it will cost you.

Questions to Ask About Particular Donors

WHAT IS HIS FAMILY MEDICAL HISTORY?

Make sure you really study the more detailed donor profile. Look for diseases like cancer and heart disease, chronic conditions like eczema and allergies, and genetic problems like dwarfism and color blindness. Some list alcoholism, and some also now list whether a donor has been exposed to CMV (cytomegalovirus). An estimated 80 percent of adults in the United States have been exposed to or infected with CMV, a member of the herpes virus family that does not manifest as sores. It is spread through casual contact in places like childcare centers, as well as during sexual contact between adults. It is generally harmless, but can be dangerous if passed to a fetus through its mother, and the baby can develop health problems as a result. Statistically, CMV is now the virus most often transmitted to a developing baby before birth. (See the sidebar later in this chapter.)

What Is CMV?

Cytomegalovirus, a member of the herpes virus family, is now thought to infect much of the world's population. It is spread through both sexual and nonsexual contact with other people, not via food or water. It is not a danger to most people unless they have an already weakened immune system, but it is a danger to pregnant women. If you are already infected with CMV when you become pregnant, you will probably pass it on to your baby in utero or through nursing, but it likely won't harm the child. However, if you are infected for the first time during your pregnancy, your fetus can be harmed. Some babies born from a recently infected mother can suffer mental and developmental problems, or hearing and visual impairment. For this reason, you should have yourself—and all donors you use, known or unknown—tested for CMV. If you have not been exposed previously to CMV, and your donor has, you could be infected during your pregnancy, and your fetus could be infected as well. All sperm banks should clearly indicate test results for CMV on their donor profiles.

WHAT IS HIS POST-THAW MOTILE SPERM COUNT?

Not all banks will tell you this. But if you can find out, it's a good bit of information to know. Multiple sperm work together to penetrate the egg, even though only one will get in and join with that egg. So the more sperm get to the egg, the better your chances to conceive. Most men average 20 to 80 million total sperm per cc, of which at least 10 million are motile (exhibiting movement). When I was told a donor I was considering had an exceptionally high sperm count and a high post-thaw motility rate, it became a main reason to choose him. A few months later I was pregnant.

More sperm banks are now specific about such stats on their websites. For example, the Midwest Sperm Bank specifies that their IUI-ready specimens contain a post-thaw quantity of 20 million sperm in a vial, with motility equal to or greater than 35 percent. PRS lists that their IUI-ready vials are guaranteed to contain 15 million motile sperm. Such statistics may be meaningless to you in the beginning of your journey. But if it takes you longer than a few months to become pregnant, they will become increasingly important. Beyond looking for eye color or education, you might find yourself asking clinic staff about motility and progression.

HAS HE PRODUCED OTHER LIVE CHILDREN? HOW MANY?

Some banks tell you this only if you ask, and others won't provide this information at all. Cathy Winks of the Sperm Bank of California says it is well known to sperm bank workers that some donors produce children quickly, and others never produce any.

So if you know a guy's been an active donor for more than a year and no one's ever become pregnant by him, I'd pick another guy right away.

WILL THE DONOR BE AVAILABLE IF I WANT MORE CHILDREN?

Most banks stop using a donor once a certain number of women (usually between four and ten) become pregnant by him. Generally, though, they will guarantee repeated use if you want to birth a sibling, but you should always check to make sure—even if you're not certain at the time that you'll ever want another child. You may need to prepay for these vials and keep them stored at the bank for several years, pending your decision to go ahead with a second child. If the bank needs to "reactivate" a donor and he is willing to come in and make more deposits, you usually have to pay an extra fee. Note that most donors are not willing to do this.

What You Should Expect from Your Sperm Bank

COURTEOUS, KNOWLEDGEABLE SERVICE

Staff should be friendly, empathetic, and willing to answer your questions. Especially when you are first starting out, it's important to have the feeling that clinic staff are on your side. It can be painful and disorienting if you are given wrong information or made to feel as though your concerns are not valid.

> We asked one clinic worker if there was any way to better our chances of having a girl over a boy. We were mostly just curious, but instead of just giving us the information we wanted, she went off on a ten-minute rant about how wonderful her boy children were. We felt belittled and humiliated, and never used their services again. —Barbara

I have dealt with several clinics and found most staff people genuinely helpful and friendly. However, as in any job, staff may forget just how profoundly their words and actions can affect those who call upon them for advice. This is compounded tenfold in a setting like a fertility clinic or sperm bank, where the emotional stakes are so high and the financial repercussions so great. If you're not happy with the service you're getting from a particular person, try not to take it personally or let it affect your conception process. Ask to speak to someone else, or do a little Web trolling to identify the favorite clinician and deal only with that person. Empower yourself to get the experience you want. However, if one bank or clinic rubs you the wrong way and you have other options, by all means exercise them. Remember, sperm banks are businesses. They depend on their clients' happiness for their continued success. And your happiness may mean less stress for you, and less stress means a better chance of conceiving.

FREQUENT UPDATES OF DONOR LISTS

If these lists are not updated every few months or so, they will likely include donors who are no longer available. Especially in this age of instant information, Web lists should be updated weekly or monthly. Most sperm banks now list whether certain donors are available in limited quality, or even, as at PRS, "extremely limited" quantity, which can mean only a few vials. Some banks now update their online donor lists hourly! This is a wonderful service for women undergoing the stressful process of picking a donor. You can check in online at midnight if you feel you need to, and make sure your chosen guy's supply is still high and that he still seems the best choice to you. Or, you can scroll through the entire list of donors again, and change your mind about him completely. To be able to do so on your own timeline, with full access to information, is very empowering.

HOURS OF OPERATION THAT ARE CONVENIENT FOR YOU
If your bank or fertility clinic is open only Monday–Friday 9–5 (and many are), this may not be convenient for you. If you unexpectedly surge on a Friday night and need to inseminate on Saturday, and you can't get an appointment or sperm, you're out of luck that month! Some fertility doctors have actually put women on drugs to regulate their cycles for no other reason than the convenience to their own schedules. It might be time to seek another option at that point.

OPENNESS TO CRITICISM
If you have a complaint about the way a bank is doing business with you, you should be able to let them know. If someone gives you incorrect information or is rude to you, you should feel comfortable addressing this. Often, if there is a real problem, you may get a free month of sperm or some other compensation. I'm not talking about suing here. Rather, just as in any other commercial exchange, you should feel empowered to express dissatisfaction and not be intimidated by the "experts." The better informed you are as a client, the easier time you will have using whatever service you choose.

Ultimately, the only expert you can count on in this process is yourself. The better educated you are, the more likely you are to feel that you, the paying customer and hopeful parent, are in control of this process.

How to Choose a Donor

Choosing a donor is one of the biggest decisions you will make along your path to parenthood. Not so many years ago, women had few choices about donor selection. Basically, they took what was available through a doctor, or used a middleman or friend to deliver fresh sperm to them. Donors were generally medical students affiliated with a doctor's clinic, and friends were often gay men. At clinics, single women and lesbians were not even allowed to inseminate, and sperm banks were barely born. Some of the earliest sperm banks in California were formed expressly so that single women and dykes could get pregnant.

These days, not only are lesbians a large percentage of many sperm banks' business, but you are likely to have a potentially overwhelming number of donors to choose from. The industry average is about 20–25 active donors, but some sperm banks have up to a hundred. When you pick a sperm bank, you are basically trusting it to provide you with a range of donors. A few of these will be desirable to you, and if all goes well, you will get pregnant by one of them.

Selecting a donor is not a decision to take lightly. So the first question you need to ask yourself is, what is the genetic makeup you want for your future child? Some things may be obvious to you. For example, you may decide you only want a Caucasian donor, or an African American. This will narrow the field considerably. But what if you want a biracial child? Or you are an unusual biracial mixture yourself and want to duplicate it? If you have a partner, would you prefer that the donor's physical appearance match hers more closely than yours? Do you want someone who is highly educated? Who has traveled extensively? Who has lots of siblings? And what if you like everything about a donor until you find out there's a history of breast cancer or eczema in his family? Do you still pick him?

Some donor profiles will seem to just jump off the page at you (hey, he's got red hair and plays the piano!), but it's also possible you'll have to really hunt for one that looks good to you. I would advise taking your time to narrow your selections to the top five, and not pin all your hopes on just one donor. That one may not be available, or his supply might run out just when you need it, and you will feel very let down.

Remember that each donor is a human being, and be realistic about what that means. For example, one friend of mine realized that she was discounting every donor in one clinic's book because "someone in his family had died." While we can make informed choices about certain family traits we wish to avoid, escaping death isn't possible. Once she clued in and realized she was making superhuman demands of her child's genetic pool, she lightened up, picked a donor, and conceived on her first try.

Her good luck might be yours too, but if you try for a while with one donor and don't get pregnant, consider switching. This can be very empowering after a period of bad luck, and you'll feel that you're giving yourself a fresh start.

Some women have described a strong adverse reaction after using a donor. Something about how their body responded just didn't seem right to them. Or they didn't like the smell of his sperm. Definitely listen to your intuition about these things, and make adjustments accordingly.

> If you are using an unknown donor, don't be afraid to switch donors if one is not working out for you. We changed three times until we finally got a keeper. —Joani

Just to play devil's advocate, I will note here that I don't believe it is really possible for you to pick a "wrong" donor and therefore have the "wrong" baby. Whatever baby you have—or even adopt—will be the right baby for you. All your preplanning for perfection can only take you so far. It's mind-boggling to consider the infinite genetic combinations that can be created from just one ejaculate and one egg. Watching women struggle for weeks with donor choices has made me wonder if it wouldn't be easier just to pick a random donor and let nature take its course. While I don't advocate a total lack of planning, I don't recommend spending fruitless hours nitpicking about donor choices if it's time to get busy inseminating. Your resulting baby will be just as perfect if you spend four or 40 hours picking a donor. Don't let indecision about finding the perfect donor prevent you from getting pregnant.

The Money Factor

Sperm Bank Costs

Helpfully, most sperm banks now list their prices on their websites. The price list shows fees for all their products and services, including donor semen, donor reactivation, supplies, and shipping.

Below is a price list from a typical sperm bank, with an explanation of the most common terms you will encounter.

REGISTRATION: $150
This is a one-time fee some banks charge for an intake. Not all sperm banks charge this, but if it is required, you have to pay it. At the time of

intake, a staff member may go over some information such as how to chart your cycles and inform you about clinic hours for sperm pickup.

HEALTH TESTS: $0–$600

Many sperm banks require that you be healthy and be able to prove it. Some ask for a minimal number of blood tests (such as proof of HIV status), but others want many more, such as tests for HTLV-1, CMV, syphilis, rubella, toxoplasmosis, Tay-Sachs disease, sickle-cell disease, and mycoureaplasma. These can become expensive. You will be charged for these tests if you have them at the clinic. If you have a regular doctor or are covered by a health plan, you would probably prefer to get them done in advance and bring in the results. Other banks ship only to doctors' offices, under the assumption that you have had these tests done by your own provider. And do check what your health insurance covers before you pay out of pocket for anything. You may be covered for more—or less—than you thought.

FOR INTRACERVICAL OR HOME INSEMINATIONS

FROZEN SEMEN: $150–$250 PER CC

A cc, or cubic centimeter, of semen is the tiny amount provided by sperm banks in little plastic vials. You may not believe that such a small amount of semen can ever get you pregnant. But each vial should contain millions and millions of sperm, more than enough to get the job done. Studies show that trying twice each month can double your chances. This means you will also double your costs—at least $300 for two vials. Note that some sperm banks charge more for the semen of men who are willing to be known to the child later in life.

FOR INTRAUTERINE PROCEDURE

PROCEDURE: $300 AND UP

INTRAUTERINE-READY SPECIMEN: $200–$250 PER 1 CC OR LESS (USUALLY .06–.08 ML)

Aside from more high-tech and expensive methods, I believe that an intrauterine (IUI) is the optimal procedure for healthy women starting out on the conception roller coaster. While there are no hard-and-fast statistics, it generally takes only half as long to get pregnant by regularly trying IUIs at a clinic or sperm bank, compared to home inseminations using just a syringe. Why?

For one thing, you know that intrauterine-ready sperm are viable. There's no opportunity for your dry ice to run out, or for the syringe to slip, or for any of the other mishaps that can occur at home. Following the procedure at the clinic, you can even look in the microscope and see an "extra" drop or two of sperm swimming with life. I was never convinced that the samples I brought home were actually capable of making me pregnant. Seeing my donor's magnified sperm so motile gave me an emotional boost and really made me believe I would soon get pregnant.

When you receive an IUI, the ejaculate is generally spun in a machine called a centrifuge to remove the active swimmers from the rest of the liquid semen. The sperm may be mixed with a solution made especially for this purpose. This concentrated solution, only about half a cc of liquid, is then fed through a tube that is passed through your cervix and into your uterus. The sperm do not have to swim through your body's fertile mucus at all. This is an advantage, since the mucus can be a difficult obstacle course for the little swimmers. In fact, by completely bypassing the trek through your vagina, the sperm get about a five-hour head start. Since frozen sperm may only live about 12 hours, this places them a lot closer to the egg at this critical time. IUI is a more expensive procedure than home insemination, but it may prove to be a lot cheaper than endless rounds of home inseminations.

Do IUIs hurt? While there is some chance of cramping, most women experience no discomfort at all. I felt a slight sensation when the tiny tube was fed through my cervix, and that was about it. It was a lot less messy than an insemination at home, and just as fast.

Some midwives are now skilled in doing intrauterine inseminations for their clients at home. Often they use a minicentrifuge, or process the sperm so that it separates from the rest of the semen. If you are thinking about using a midwife for your birth, you may want to ask her if she is qualified to help you inseminate as well. That way you can combine the comfort and intimacy of being in your own home with the greater effectiveness of the IUI method.

If you have a clinic insemination, ask that you be told exactly what is happening during the procedure, find out whether your partner or a friend can help push the plunger, and make sure the room is heated to your liking. If it's chilly, make sure you are provided with a blanket before clinic staff leave the room. Otherwise, you may lie there alone, half-naked, and shivering while you wait for your allotted half hour to pass. Let clinic staff know in advance that you'll want to relax in the room awhile. Give those expensive sperm every chance you can to swim up as far into your body as possible.

FOR INTRACERVICAL PROCEDURE

PROCEDURE: $300 AND UP

SPERM: $200 AND UP

An intracervical is like an intrauterine, except that the semen is not deposited as far up as your uterus. It will be placed just on the other side of your cervical opening, or right at the opening. An intracervical may be performed because your cervix is partially closed, and the intrauterine tube just won't go any farther. Despite the fact that an intracervical may be less effective than an intrauterine, this is the procedure that finally got me pregnant. Some clinics use the term *intracervical* to mean any kind of insemination that isn't an IUI, including home insemination without even a speculum.

It All Adds Up

Yes, trying to get pregnant can get very expensive! Besides the costs listed above, you may be spending money on costly fertility drugs. *Getting pregnant with frozen sperm will cost an average of $400–$700 per cycle if you are inseminating at home, or $500–$1000 per cycle if you are using the services of a clinic or bank for procedures such as IUI.* In addition, there may be extra fees for weeknight, weekend, or Sunday hours at a clinic, which you may end up paying if your cycle or schedule requires you to inseminate at those times. You may also need to have sperm shipped or stored, if you do not live near a clinic, or the clinic of your choice. So you must factor in the cost of renting or shipping a liquid-nitrogen tank from the bank for storing the sperm to keep them cold enough. You will also have to pay to ship the tank back to the bank. Women who bring sperm home from a bank must buy a cooler to store it in, as well as dry ice, each cycle, to keep it cold. And since dry ice loses at least half its volume each day, you may have to buy several batches of it each month you are trying. Other monthly expenses include syringes, and of course, your ovulation predictor kits.

True, you may be one of the lucky gals who gets pregnant the first time. However, you should realistically plan on spending $500–$1,000 for your first cycle, including lab work and intake fees, and $400–$700 for each cycle thereafter. Trying to get pregnant twice a cycle may double your chances, but it will also probably double your costs. The high expense of getting pregnant can add tremendously to the stress of trying to get pregnant. When your finances start to dwindle, take a month or two off to recoup.

I frequently read, on online bulletin boards, women carping about the tremendous costs involved in trying to conceive. But remember, gals, the cost of conceiving your baby is only the very beginning of the costs associated with having a child. If you can't afford to GET pregnant, how will you afford a child? Keep in mind that if you plan to pay for day care or preschool for your child a year or two down the line, you will be looking at costs of at least $800 a month, if not significantly more. My daughter's preschool tab came to a thousand bucks a month, and her "after-school" care for two hours after public school each day is still $400 a month. The few thousand dollars I spent trying to conceive my daughter is now long forgotten, and it pales in comparison to the more than $50K I've probably spent on childcare in the years since. If you can't afford $400 a month for sperm to make a baby, examine your finances, or at least your financial priorities, immediately.

Insurance

Some women are lucky enough to have their fertility services covered in full by their health insurance. Others can claim partial coverage. Most women aren't able to claim much. But every policy is different—ask in advance, so you know what's up, and you may be able to upgrade or change coverage completely to get a break. To avoid being denied coverage, you may have to claim that you are unable to conceive "naturally," rather than say you are a lesbian. Some insurance packages cover the services of a fertility clinic but not the sperm. Or you may just feel more comfortable paying for the services of the sperm bank of your choice, even if you have insurance through a provider such as an HMO. Of course, if you don't have insurance, you will end up paying for everything anyway.

*Most insurance companies don't cover "infertility treatment,"
which is what artificial insemination is classified as, but most do
cover the rest of your maternity expenses—i.e., prenatal exams,
hospital or birthing center delivery, etc. Just get the best deal you
can. Remember to check out your insurance company's preap-
proval clauses. I was moments from delivery and on the phone
with the damned insurance people—they called the hospital
when the first paperwork reached them, and wondered what the
heck was happening! Arghhhh! What did they think all those
prenatal expenses were for, fun? Dealing with them between
contractions was not enjoyable! —Marissa*

Trying to Get Pregnant at Home

Some Things You Will Need for Each Home Insemination

- A small, six-pack-sized cooler in which to carry the sperm, and an
  adequate supply of dry ice
- A speculum for isolating your cervix (if you choose to use one)
- A flashlight for examining your cervix
- A needleless syringe for insemination—have a few of these on
  hand in case you need more than one per insemination cycle
- A towel to place under your buttocks to absorb spillage of semen
- Disposable latex gloves for the inseminator to use if she's squea-
  mish about touching semen

*Our sperm bank was in California, so we pretty much had to guess
when we'd be ovulating and needing the sperm shipped. If we were
early by more than forty-eight hours, we had to keep the sperm on
dry ice, and we had a hard time finding that in the town where we
lived. At first we didn't tell Baskin Robbins why we needed the dry
ice we'd ask for every month. But after several months of this, they
knew what we were doing and were cheering us on. —Angela*

*When we had our sperm delivered, were we ever surprised to see
a cute baby butch lesbian driver handing over the goods. She
looked knowingly at the box marked "medical supplies," smiled,
said "good luck," and drove off! —Beverly*

How to Try at Home

Many lesbians, particularly those in couples, prefer to try to become pregnant at home initially. If you are using semen from a sperm bank, you will have to thaw it according to the clinic's instructions. The most common procedure is to set the vial of frozen semen in warm (not hot) water for about five minutes until it thaws to room temperature and a runny consistency. The objective is not to thaw it as quickly as possible, but to thaw it gently, so the sperm come back to their optimum motility. Some women prefer to thaw the vial under their arm or otherwise next to their body, since this temperature will stay more consistent. Wait until it has completely thawed, and turned to a runny, more liquid consistency, before using it. Note that the vials are extremely cold when they come out of the tank or cooler and you may need to use a glove to handle them at first.

It's important to pay close attention to the thawing process. You don't want to use semen that is still cold or has defrosted from a too-slow thaw. If it has been sitting around on the bathroom counter for longer than an hour or two, it most likely won't be viable.

You have about an hour total from the time you begin to thaw a vial until the time you should inseminate. Other sperm facts to know: You cannot refreeze a vial if it thaws, or keep fresh sperm at home in a regular freezer. Keeping sperm frozen requires a *much*

When using the services of a fertility OB/GYN, you might be asked to attend one or more counseling sessions. This is considered a routine procedure for both straight and gay couples, particularly if you are using the services of a sperm bank. It may rub you the wrong way to have to do this, since you probably have already put so much thought into this process. If you can show that you have already thought through many of the issues involved, you may be able to have these sessions waived.

colder temperature than that of your refrigerator or freezer. Remember also to keep your cooler or tank tightly closed and out of the sun. Some women wrap their coolers in a towel to help keep them cold. Having done an insemination at home several times using a cooler and without becoming pregnant, I advise you to use a liquid-nitrogen tank instead. It stays colder for longer, and you won't have to worry about the dry ice evaporating. You'll lose the use of the sperm if this happens—as it did to me once.

For the actual insemination, the preferred method is to use a needle-less syringe to draw up the sperm. (The stereotypical turkey baster will not work with the tiny amounts of sperm you buy from a bank. It's just a laughable urban legend that any dyke can become pregnant with a turkey baster.) Some women simply lie back and squirt the goods in, letting nature take its course from there. Others prop up their lower body, using pillows to angle themselves. Place the syringe in your vagina gently and as far back as is comfortable. Remember to depress the syringe slowly.

Syringes

It may be difficult to find a place where you can purchase the thin needleless syringes that are best used for insemination. If you are using a sperm bank and plan to inseminate at home, the bank will probably supply 1 cc syringes. If you are not using a sperm bank, you may have a hard time buying syringes in stores and may have to order them online. While some drugstore and medical supply companies do stock them, you usually need a doctor's prescription to purchase syringes. However, most national drugstore chains sell something called a medicine applicator, used to give medicine to children orally, for under $3. A medicine applicator is essentially a thick, needleless syringe and will do the job quite nicely. Some pharmacies even give them out for free! It is ironic that a forbidden syringe can be repackaged as an "oral syringe" (the Walgreens kit even comes with a cleaning brush to scrub it out with) and sold next to diapers and baby bottles in the drugstore. If only they knew!

Speculums

Check women's health centers, local midwives, or Planned Parenthood for speculums. Plastic reusable speculums can also be mail-ordered from Awakenings Birth Services in San Francisco. See the resources chapter for details.

Some women use a speculum (plastic is much more comfortable than metal) so their partner or friend can see their cervix. If you've opened the speculum and can't see the cervix, you need to adjust the speculum until you do. This can be uncomfortable, so do it gently. You may need a flashlight to help see the cervix, since the inside of your body is dark! If your insemination timing is right, the cervix should ideally appear open and a bit wet with a clearish mucus. Some women's cervixes produce so much mucus when they're fertile that it will be oozing out. This is a good sign of fertility, so don't worry that it will block the entrance to your uterus—the sperm will swim right through it!

If you are doing the insemination yourself, be careful not to get overly excited and drop, or accidentally depress, the syringe; the last thing you want is to shoot the sperm across the room. This actually happened to friends of mine! It may be a good idea to have another friend present to hold the flashlight. If you are using a speculum, you can check to make sure that at least some of the semen is coated on or around the cervix, though you don't want to aim inside the cervix—that can cause infection. The syringe should be depressed slowly and steadily, and withdrawn the same way. Be as careful as you can not to pull the speculum out quickly. This can hurt you, and it could cause you to lose quite a bit of the semen you've just inseminated. Some spillage from the vagina is inevitable in any insemination, but a speculum will cause more to be lost. Don't worry—it will take you a try or two to get comfortable with this procedure.

The most embarrassing moment of my pregnancy was when an old girlfriend of my partner's came over and showed us how to place the semen inside me. Of course, I had to "assume the position" for her, and I had never even met her before! —Nadine

Many women like to elevate their bottom on pillows or rest it against a wall for twenty minutes or more after insemination, to allow the sperm a better shot at swimming up into the uterus. This is probably a good idea, though I've also heard stories about women inseminating themselves in their car and then driving off to a meeting, and still ending up pregnant. Go figure.

There is certainly an intimacy about trying at home that cannot be duplicated at even the most well-meaning clinic. This is especially so if you are a couple—the nonbiological partner will feel much more involved if she's actually the one doing the insemination. It may also be nice to try to incorporate lovemaking into the ritual, though I found I was usually too tense to have sex after or before insemination. Studies show that orgasms actually help suck sperm up into the uterus, so sex could help your insemination odds. Remember not to use lube if you decide to include sex play as part of the insemination—and make sure not to expose the other woman or women present to the sperm. Rumor has it that several lesbian partners have gotten pregnant this way.

> Sex after insemination was wonderful! As an incest survivor I felt this was a way of putting men in their proper place. They served a purpose in the creation of a baby without having to be directly involved. Very freeing for me! —Estela

Since some midwives are now qualified to do intrauterine inseminations, at-home IUIs may soon become the preferred method of trying to conceive. Midwives may recommend the use of sperm cups or other tricks of the trade. You have the right to choose to use any, all, or none.

Trying at home can be romantic at first, but using the services of a professional clinic can be more effective in the long term.

Because trying at home can be as intimate as you like, feel free to plan a conception ceremony for your first try. This might include a blessing, candles, and poetry. If you take more than a few cycles to conceive, however, you may find that you bother less with these things and get down to business more quickly. Do try to lie still, with your bottom slightly elevated, for up to an hour afterward. Make sure you pee before you start the insemination, and if you're doing self-insemination, make sure you have everything you need close by and handy for your rest period afterward.

> We have a seven-month-old girl conceived on the third try. On that attempt we dimmed the lights and brought out special items from our two other children. We spent thirty minutes in the doctor's office, with my partner lying upside down on the table with her hips raised and me giving her those items one by one. —Toni

> We did all the right things the first time around and made that try special...and we didn't get pregnant. By try six we were watching Jeopardy! while inseminating. And try fourteen was all-around irritating, with bad scheduling and a hectic day and rotten traffic, and we were sure we had the timing all wrong—and that's when we got pregnant. It was about as romantic as a root canal. —Rebecca

In my own case, after three or four months of trying, I became convinced that there was no way I was ever going to become pregnant at home with frozen sperm. There were just too many variables, such as whether I had thawed the sperm properly, or whether a dwindling supply of dry ice had kept the sperm viable. It was actually a relief to begin going in for my monthly intrauterines at the clinic, because the onus shifted from my own capabilities to theirs. I didn't need to have semen sitting around the house—it could stay at the clinic till I was ready. Perhaps, if I had conceived very quickly, this would never have become an issue. But after trying at home for several months, I was ready for a change. At Rainbow Flag's clinic I was even able to view some of the sperm sample under the microscope afterward, and watch the last few little sperm swim crazily around on a slide. It was a relief to know that not only had the goods thawed properly, but most of them were at that very moment dashing merrily along inside me in search of that ever-elusive egg.

Some fertility clinics can store your bank-bought semen at their facilities until you're ready to use it. Some require you to keep it yourself until your insemination day, or pick it up from the bank and bring it directly over. The clinician or fertility specialist will examine it when you're ready to inseminate and make sure the sperm are viable. In some cases, the clinic will suggest you use a different donor or a different bank altogether. Negotiating all these tactical maneuvers is part of your insemination learning process.

Other Options

Using an Anonymous Donor with Fresh Sperm, through a Middleman

Although using an anonymous donor through a middleman was the way many lesbians got pregnant in the pre-AIDS era, this practice is no longer in favor. Health considerations dictate that this method is not safe, as you know nothing about the donor or his health—physical or mental. Legally it is also not sound, since it is relatively easy for the donor to find out whom he has impregnated.

Sex with a Man

More lesbians and bisexual women than you might expect try to get pregnant by having sex with a man. Or at least they think about it. There's something so tempting about the thought of two warm bodies joining together in the magical act of conceiving a child. It can be so much more appealing than lying spread-eagled under bright lights on a clinic table. Unlike alternative insemination, sex is inexpensive, and if you like sex with men, it can be enjoyable. Of course, many women find this thought utterly unappealing. And the health and legal risks involved in conceiving this way are numerous. The man may have an STI, or CMV infection. And most chillingly, the courts will consider him the legal father of your child if he claims paternity. Conceivably, this could give him equal access to your long-awaited child!

Lawyers and healthcare practitioners wince at the notion of a lesbian considering sex with a man—particularly one you don't know well—to get pregnant. But many women do it, and end up having perfectly healthy children, and they never have to see the father again. (Read lesbian writer Carole Maso's book *The Room Lit by Roses* for a first-hand account of this approach.) Other women decide that the man they are inseminating with will be known to the child as the father. (See "The Father Factor," earlier in this chapter.)

In my own frustration at not getting pregnant quickly with frozen sperm, I occasionally contemplated flying off to some small town somewhere, or even to another country, to have casual sex a few times during my ovulation week. In fact, I was convinced that I would get pregnant immediately this way. If you are single, it may be very tempting to try this.

On the other hand, if you have a lover, she may have a serious issue with your sleeping with some dude to get knocked up. And really, who can blame her!

Chapter 5

Surviving the Roller Coaster—
Ten Tips to Keep You Sane

If there's one thing I learned from the roller coaster, it's that there are no guarantees...and that it's really important to find the humor in it all. —Karin

Only women who are intentionally trying to get pregnant (and paying lots of money to do so, besides!) can appreciate the madness of this process. The rest of the world will have no idea what you're going through. Even if you try for a year or two, people won't comprehend the stress you're feeling. Only those who have lived through it are truly aware of the emotional and physical roller-coaster ride that trying to conceive will throw us onto, and the two-week life cycle that our lives suddenly revolve around. I'm here to tell you that unless you get pregnant on your first try, you will most likely be plunged into this world of emotional upheaval. There's no easy way to survive this time, and it won't end until you get pregnant, but the good news is that it *will* end. This may be hard to believe as you read this chapter. I myself remember thinking that this roller coaster was now a permanent condition, and I was going to be riding it forever!

I've always believed in the power of distraction. Go to lots of movies. Go for long, energetic walks. Decide to reorganize your bookshelves or do some early Christmas shopping. Every time you start to talk—or even think—about the baby thing, actively change the subject. —Kaia

Plan to not be pregnant, and think about the next try. So either you're all prepared for the disappointment, or you get to be surprised and do happy dances about how there won't be a "next" time. And don't do a pregnancy test too early—you don't want to get a negative result and your period on the same day. A definite downer! —Mary

Let me reassure you that once you conceive, you'll look back on this time and say, "Oh, I guess it wasn't so bad." This may seem unbelievable now, but when you're fighting off morning sickness or feeling that baby move around in your belly, the awful months of trying will have slipped almost completely out of your head. And when your baby is born, you might just decide you love the first one so much that a second would be a good idea. Yes, you might one day willingly submit to this process all over again!

But for now—some tips on how to take care of yourself, and your relationship, so that you can survive this most stressful of times.

1. Take Care of Yourself First

Self-care is absolutely the most important part of this whole process. This is a time of unbelievable stress for most of us, and there won't be many people around who understand how trying it all is. Therefore, do everything you can to be gentle with yourself now. Get enough sleep, eat well, indulge in a monthly massage, take long baths, and commune with whatever Goddess you believe in. Don't give in to drinking too much alcohol, or other unhealthy ways of dealing with stress. Once you can relax as much as possible about this process, it will become easier to bear. At the same time, be gentle with your lover if you have one, especially if you are doing this together. Trying to get pregnant is a hard thing for couples, and many break up during this time. Don't let wanting a baby destroy your partnership.

If you are doing this as a couple, it is essential to have a rock-solid relationship. Our relationship always came first and was never compromised by our attempts to get pregnant. —Margie

2. Understand That It's Probably Going to Take a While

Sure, some people get lucky the first time, and we all hope that it's going to be us. I have friends who have conceived on their first try and are convinced it should be that easy for everyone. Others have the humility to know that they were just lucky. For the rest of us, surviving this really difficult time becomes a bit easier if we can understand that, especially with frozen sperm, conception usually takes at least a few tries. That's why I always recommend trying at home a time or two just for the experience, and then stepping up the effectiveness of your methods, perhaps with an intrauterine at the clinic.

> My girlfriend and I are using the IUI method with the help of an infertility doctor and Clomid. When we first started planning to have a baby, we never thought it would be this much work. No one told us about the time involved looking through donor catalogs, trying to find that "perfect donor" and then living through those long two week intervals that our lives seemed to be spent in. We got through it by thinking of how worth it all this would all be in the end. —Sarah

Additionally, you may want to wait a few months before you announce to everyone that you're trying—otherwise, well-wishers will ask you every month if you've succeeded. People probably don't realize that, instead of appearing supportive, their inquiries can be irritating.

> If you don't want everyone asking you every month if you are finally pregnant, limit the people who know you're trying. We told many people, and every month it was very painful each time we'd get asked again if it happened yet. —Denise

3. Realize That Your Life Will Now Be Divided into Two-Week Cycles

> The anxiety of not knowing if I'm pregnant is unbelievable. I never imagined it would be like this. The two-week waiting period is driving us nuts! —Leila

Sure, weeks used to flow by without much notice, but that's all changed now. Once you start trying to conceive a baby, every month of your life will go something like this:

Stage 1

You'll get your period and cry for a day. You'll bleed for a few days, then call the sperm bank (or your donor) and let them know you will need their services again this month. You will start taking your temperature and watching for signs of fertile mucus. You will become more agitated each day. You'll pee on a few ovulation sticks and overanalyze their readings. When all signs are a go that you're on the brink of popping out your egg, you'll make an appointment with the sperm bank or donor. You will inseminate, either at home, trying to be romantic, or at the clinic or doctor's office, up on the examining table. You will tremble with excitement at the prospect that this could be the time, even while you are marveling at the inhumanity of the whole damn process.

Stage 2

Now that you are inseminated, you will anxiously take your temperature every day to see if it stays high or falls. You will become a hypochondriac examining every sign of possible early pregnancy or PMS. Confusingly, their symptoms are very similar, so you won't be sure what to believe. Your girlfriend will come to loathe the thermometer beeping first thing in the morning. You will drive your friends crazy asking, "Do you think I could be pregnant this time?" You will stop drinking alcohol and avoid the hot tub, "just in case." You will be sure you might be, could be, probably are pregnant this time. Then after a few days of high-stakes anxiety, you will bleed, you will cry, and the whole grueling process will begin again.

4. Keep Believing It Could Happen Anytime

After eight years together, my partner and I decided to have a baby. We decided to try for a year, but after eleven months of taking my temperature, checking those lovely cervical fluids, arguing over whether the blue line on the ovulation test stick was "blue enough," we were still not pregnant. It is such a trying

road when month after month you obsess about something so important. Before we went in for our twelfth and last insemination I learned some devastating family news and decided I wouldn't try that time. My partner encouraged me to go, knowing I would regret it later if I didn't. Two weeks later we were shopping, buying a box of tampons and a pregnancy test, knowing we'd need one of them the next day. And now I sit holding my four-month-old son, the most incredibly gorgeous baby to ever grace this planet. I guess my message is to never give up. Keep the faith; you never know what miracles await you.
—Wendy

That story pretty much says it all. I can't absolutely guarantee that you'll conceive any more than I can predict a major earthquake, but I can tell you that Wendy's story is typical. The time I conceived, I was convinced that it couldn't possibly happen that month. But it did for me, and it could for you, too.

It's really important to know that if you don't get pregnant the first time and have to try again, it's not because you didn't do all the right things at the right time. Don't blame yourselves! Don't waste a moment's stress thinking, "If only we'd done X first" or "If only we'd done Y second" or "If only we'd stood on our heads every second Tuesday." You have to step back and let nature take its course, which is a good first lesson in parenting: you are not 100 percent in control anymore! —Ruth

5. Find Support Wherever You Can

I lived in gay mecca, San Francisco, when I was trying to conceive, and I'm a pretty well-connected person. But I still felt as though I was reinventing the wheel every menstrual cycle. The fact is, even with the gayby boom in full force, trying to conceive is a tremendously isolating experience. You will probably feel as if you are the only dyke in the world who has ever gone through this. As supportive as they may be in the beginning, your friends will soon get bored with your monthly angst. So you will have to look elsewhere: Start with friends of friends who are trying (call them, even if they're strangers, because they soon may be your best friends). Then check online bulletin boards and support groups. (See the resources chapter of this book for some starting points online.) There are sites specifically for single women, like the Yahoo board "singlemomsbychoice." These gals offer moral support and good medical advice on fertility drugs. In some cities, there may be "insemination support groups" specifically for lesbians, possibly offered through the practices of lesbian midwives. Even just finding one sympathetic person at the sperm bank who remembers your name and empathizes with what you are going through will make the whole process much more humanizing.

You may find that some of your childless dyke friends have no frame of reference for your entire, all-consuming prepregnancy experience, and they may be unsympathetic. Other dyke friends may be seasoned "aunties" well versed in the experience of their lesbian mom friends. And you may find yourself bonding, in ways you wouldn't have imagined previously, with straight women who are trying to conceive. Since many of them have had children or are trying to, they may relate to your struggle immediately. Sexual boundaries may melt before your eyes. During my pregnancy, it was one or two dyke friends, my online chat board, and a whole bevy of straight customers at the bookshop I owned at the time who gave me the most backup. Get support wherever you can, and don't be afraid to reach out for it from unlikely sources.

6. Don't Hang Out with Unsupportive People

It's exhausting enough having to educate everyone you care about, so don't waste energy on the cads. I had to learn this the hard way, during my first trimester, when I went out to dinner with dyke friends of my then girlfriend. As sick as I was feeling those first few months, it was all I could do to drag myself out to the restaurant to meet these new gals. Somehow, during their line of very invasive questioning about the whole ordeal, my girlfriend at the time let slip that my sex drive was way down. If you talk to other pregnant women, you hear that this is very common. Weeks of surging hormones and throwing up take their toll, after all. But one of the gals launched into a huge explanation of why she thought my sex drive had decreased, none of it supportive or well informed. Because I already felt vulnerable, and didn't know these women well, I was humiliated. There is no room for this kind of hurt in anyone's pregnancy. You will be emotionally volatile enough without acquaintances merrily spewing forth their uninformed ideas. Pitch people like this right out of your life!

Other types to avoid are people who think parenthood is for the birds, people who hate children, people who have a disturbing analysis of why you aren't getting pregnant, and anyone who thinks queers shouldn't have kids. Remember, too, that relatives who initially may not be supportive of your desire to parent will likely rally once the baby arrives.

7. Expect Your Body to Freak Out, but Try Not to Obsess So Much That You Really Flip Out

Yes, expect all sorts of disconcerting things to happen to you from the stress of trying to get pregnant. For me, my usually regular 28-to-30-day menstrual cycle started jumping anywhere from 26 to 34 days. Some months I'd have fertile mucus, others I wouldn't. I got a weird infection in my mouth. I broke out with zits. I thought I just might be going insane. My friends thought I was, too. Relax; all this is (unfortunately) normal.

> Prepare yourself to become obsessive. You'll be drinking cough syrup, brewing up horrible-tasting teas, and doing your ovulation tests in the office restroom. —Zada

8. Take Time Out When You Need It

If you feel that you are at the edge of a nervous breakdown, take time out. Skip a month or two to regain your sanity, your finances, or both. It will be extremely hard to stop in the middle of this process and take a breather. You will feel your biological clock ticking and wonder each time you miss a month, "Could this have been the time?" Perhaps. But your body and brain need an occasional rest from the tremendous strain of this whole process. Maybe you could justify the break by skipping the astrological signs you don't want your kid to be born under, or come up with another reason, equally valid. Some studies have shown that women who actively engage in stress reduction, meditation, and visualization became pregnant sooner. Even if you don't believe those findings, it's still important to keep your body and mind in the best shape you can during this process.

9. Indulge in Parenting Books, Magazines, and Websites, and Visit Playgrounds

Start learning about and enjoying the world of parenting, even though you're not pregnant yet. Read parenting books and magazines to get connected to the issues of parenting. Where can you find some good ones? Try your nearest independent or feminist bookstore, to start. Subscribe to a parenting magazine like *Mothering, Hip Mama, BrainChild,* or *Parenting* to bring a little parental energy into your home every month. And if you start reading these publications now, you'll be all the more informed later about things like potty training, setting limits, and ear infections. Certainly all the pictures of cute kids in fashionable togs will cheer you up as you wonder what your own little tyke will look like. Especially if you're feeling that parenthood is all just a shaky dream, display these publications proudly on your coffee table, so you'll remember, and everyone else will realize, that you're serious about this endeavor. There are also online gay/lesbian magazines and sites like www.ProudParenting.com.

You might join an organization like Family Pride Coalition, an advocacy group for queer parents, to help you feel connected to the glbtq parenting community. And take a friend's kids to that local playground you're longing to spend time in. You'll likely end up talking to someone who's got some hot new fertility tip, or who knows a pregnant lesbian couple she can introduce you to. Even if you just end up chasing toddlers around in a game of tag, you'll have a great time, and it'll help you remember why you're trying to conceive.

10. Reevaluate Your Process as Necessary

The conception roller coaster has many twists and turns along the way, so don't be rigid about anything. Here are some of the things I pondered and then changed my mind about over the course of the year it took me to get pregnant: Sleep with a guy or use frozen sperm? Use a known or unknown donor? Which donor to pick? Change donors after a few unsuccessful tries? Inseminate at home or at the clinic? Progress from simple vaginal inseminations to more expensive (and more effective) intrauterines? Inseminate once per cycle, or twice? Or even more often? Change sperm banks altogether? Take fertility drugs or not? Which ones? For how long? Most women go through a whole litany of decisions as they wind their way toward becoming pregnant. The little line you draw in the sand, beyond which you're not willing to go, will move with time. Allow it to.

Final Survival Tip

Punch anyone who asks you, month after month, "So, are you pregnant yet?" (Just kidding—sort of!)

6

Why Am I Not Pregnant Yet? Obstacles on the Path to Parenthood

What Constitutes Infertility?

The term *infertile* has been applied traditionally to women who are unable to conceive after one year of trying through sexual intercourse. Lesbians often are routed to "infertility" services because they aren't in a heterosexual relationship and can't get pregnant the old-fashioned way. This can be offensive to lesbians who feel they are indeed fertile and healthy but simply lack ready access to sperm. They may not want to go to a clinic, or undergo physical or psychological testing, or they balk at even having to buy donor sperm. Those who eschew the clinic route entirely may ask a friend to donate his sperm, then they inseminate at home once or twice, and find they get pregnant quite easily. Why, then, is everyone making such a big deal about trying to get pregnant, they might wonder. I understand this position, and I wish pregnancy were so easy for every dyke out there. But, of course, it's not.

It's certainly unfair to be labeled "infertile" just because we don't have ready access to sperm. For a healthy woman under 35, setting off on the path to pregnancy by being pushed into infertility services is a poor start; and it creates a skewed view of conception. You might need to use a fertility clinic for insurance or legal purposes, or because you can't find a doctor outside the clinic to work with shipped frozen sperm. If this is how you need to go about getting pregnant, understand your own goals going in, and make these services work for you. Don't let the medicalization of your pregnancy overtake you and your partner. With luck, you will achieve your dream pregnancy, sooner rather than later.

On the other hand, there are millions of lesbians of childbearing age in the United States. If only a fraction of these women try to conceive, that's still hundreds of thousands who may actually need fertility services. Why? Lesbians sometimes wait later in life to try to get pregnant, so they are less fertile when they start. Or they may have previously undetected problems with their fertility—problems discovered only after a year or two of trying to conceive. Lesbians also tend to inseminate only once a month, usually with frozen sperm. Again, this lowers your odds of conception compared with a sexually active hetero couple having sex with fresh sperm. Some lesbian midwives recommend trying to inseminate multiple times each month before you self-diagnose infertility. But even among healthy straight women having lots of intercourse, about a quarter need help conceiving. So for lesbians that figure can't help but be higher.

On the path to pregnancy there are often many detours. One of the hardest to deal with is the growing realization that, because you don't seem to be getting pregnant, something might be wrong. Everyone who tries to get pregnant hopes conception will take place quickly, but we all know realistically that it can take a while. This may be especially true for women who are over 35 or using frozen sperm. You know by now that riding the conception roller coaster is a common experience. So you may not question why you can't seem to get pregnant when everyone you know is pushing around a baby carriage. Even if you wanted to consult with someone sooner, many infertility doctors won't even see you unless you've tried for a year.

> We've found that most doctors don't want to do invasive procedures unless there is a good reason to suspect there is a problem. I would talk to your doctor about getting some testing done earlier on rather than waiting a year. Make sure he or she understands the expense and emotional trauma you are going through every month. I work with physicians and think many will modify their usual year's wait if you make a strong case. —Lynda

If you're trying to conceive at home with the help of a sperm bank, you might not even know about the possibility of fertility drugs. Most banks do not mention them until you bring them up. I think they're used to women taking a while to conceive using their services, and of course their profits depend on your continued business. Additionally, if you are not interacting with the bank except to order sperm, they have no reason to advise you. So aside from requiring basic health tests, they may not push for more intervention. Remember, you need to be a highly informed consumer right from the beginning of this process.

The Next Step

After eight months to a year, the frustration level for many women is past the boiling point. You will be asking yourself every day what could possibly be wrong. Why am I not getting pregnant? What can I do about it? If you haven't done so already, get a thorough checkup. Examine your eating habits and your consumption of alcohol, coffee, cigarettes, and marijuana. Are you running yourself ragged with work, family, and community commitments? Try to slow down a little. Stress is a known factor in infertility.

The next step is to ask your regular ob/gyn to recommend a reproductive endocrinologist, or RE. These are specialists who have seen many women with fertility problems and know what to look for, what tests to do, and what treatments you may need. They are much more aggressive than regular doctors about offering up-to-date suggestions for tests and procedures.

What Could Be Wrong?

Many medical problems can interfere with a woman's ability to conceive and carry a healthy baby to term. These include uterine fibroids, endometriosis, and blocked fallopian tubes. Endometriosis in particular can be a stumbling block to pregnancy. It's a disease that often causes pain but may go unnoticed until fertility questions come up. The

All women who have problems conceiving should consult a fertility specialist called a reproductive endocrinologist, and not rely on their regular ob/gyn.

—Leland Traiman, Director, Rainbow Flag Health Services and Sperm Bank condition occurs when some of the tissue that normally lines the uterus grows elsewhere in the body, particularly around or on the ovaries.

> *I have endometriosis and have been trying to get pregnant for a while. Information regarding endo and pregnancy is very confusing. Every doctor I saw gave me a different answer for everything. And my nurse practitioner told me I will never get pregnant with endo (even with it removed) unless I do in vitro. But I called an infertility clinic and they said they see women with endo get pregnant all the time. I think you really have to be willing to read a lot of material on your own, ask a lot of questions, and be an advocate for yourself. —Beverly*

You may even want to make sure that you are actually ovulating. Charting your temperature can help determine this.

> *I was charting my temperatures and noticed that they never went up, which they should if you are ovulating. I called the doctor and she told me to come in for a progesterone test. Turns out my progesterone was too low and I wasn't ovulating. So I started taking Clomid to help me ovulate. —Enid*

A good RE will leave no stone unturned on the road to getting you pregnant. Of course, what you can afford depends on your income and the type of medical coverage you have. But you should always feel that your doctor is empathetic to your particular medical situation, that she

---

His Sperm Are Not for You!

If you have used the same donor for some time, with no results, you should consider switching. Your donor's sperm count might be too low, or a common factor called "immunologic incompatibility" might be to blame. This simply means that your donor's sperm are not compatible with your body chemistry. It's now known that half of all infertility problems in hetero couples are traced directly to the man. Learn to let go of your "perfect donor," and try some different sperm. Getting pregnant might depend upon it.

---

keeps you informed of your treatment options, and that she deals with you in an open and nondiscriminatory way. If you have any doubts about whether your doctor is being as aggressive as you would like with treatments, or if you feel you (or your partner) are not being treated in a fair manner, it is best to raise the issue, or switch doctors.

> *I had fertility problems and ended up getting a hysterosalpingogram (an X-ray examination of the uterus and fallopian tubes that are injected with dye to tell whether there are blockages in the tubes), which was a rather unpleasant procedure. I couldn't see the monitor, I didn't know what was happening, and they wouldn't let my partner into the room. I was told my tubes were blocked and I would need laparoscopic surgery to clear it up. We decided from that point on that we needed to present a united front and would only accept treatment from doctors who treated us respectfully individually and as a couple. —Maureen*

If trying to conceive is itself stressful, you can imagine how hard all these added problems make it feel. Adding together doctor appointments, treatments, and inseminations, you may truly feel that your attempts to get pregnant are ruling your life.

> *Medical intervention is expensive and hard to deal with since you have to go to the doctor some seven times over two weeks for ultrasounds, consultations, and inseminations. It's very time-consuming and extremely stressful. —Tara*

> *I found that health insurance for infertility treatments is a big issue for many lesbians. I had insurance that covered my visits with my reproductive endocrinologist and surgery for endometriosis, but nothing else. I had to switch insurers and then found that not even a consultant appointment was covered. I pay for procedures out of pocket and just spent more than $400 in fertility drugs this month. —Jane*

Friends may think you are crazy to go through so much in the quest for a child, and it may be hard to relate to anyone who hasn't been through a similar ordeal. You and your partner may find yourselves increasingly cut off from the community as you grapple painfully with this heartbreaking condition.

Yet, it can also be empowering to feel at last that you know what is wrong, and that you are doing something productive about it. While fertility problems may represent a detour, it is certainly not the end of the road for many women. Try to find a few sympathetic, knowledgeable people to share your problems with, even if it means joining a support group like RESOLVE, which is primarily for straight women. There hasn't been much attention paid to the plight of the infertile lesbian, but luckily this is starting to change. Growing support within the lesbian community, including online message boards, can help alleviate the fear, shock, and isolation of this problem. E-mail majordomo@queernet.org to subscribe to QueerNet's lesbian infertility list. There are also special boards on more general parenting sites like www.babycenter.com that specifically deal with lesbians trying to conceive via Clomid and other fertility drugs. You'll be comforted to find a whole community of lesbians going through the same thing you are. There are also numerous books on the topic of infertility—albeit generally from a straight perspective. *Inconceivable: A Woman's Triumph over Despair and Statistics*, by Julia Indichova, is one I like.

> *No one can understand what we've been going through. Total strangers feel that they can comment on why I'm not getting pregnant. Some lesbians ask why, if I want a baby so badly, I don't just adopt.* —Donna

> *A friend actually asked me why my partner didn't get pregnant instead. While that might work for some couples, we are not interchangeable. For one thing, she's butch and has no desire to be pregnant. This is my dream, and I'm not done dreaming it.*
> —Lindsay

> *Having friends with whom I can share all the woes of infertility has proved vital in keeping my sanity during this process. When I went for my latest insemination a friend of mine who'd also had infertility problems came with me and brought her seven-week-old baby. When I had my IUI, which I found painful, my friend put her little boy in my arms, and I held him while the insemination took place. I figure if he can't bring me good luck, no one can.*
> —Aubrey

None of my friends understand how badly I want to become pregnant, and how ashamed I am that I can't. —Nicolette

Alternative Treatments for Infertility

I tried for nine months to get pregnant, and my doctor was not very encouraging, since he felt my chances were poor. I finally got pregnant after going to a Chinese herbalist. Don't believe everything a doctor tells you, and by all means seek "alternative" treatment. It may make all the difference. —Caroline

Before you take fertility drugs, there are other options for increasing your fertility to consider. Many women try acupuncture or herbs, practice meditation or Traditional Chinese Medicine (TCM), and even drink specially brewed teas. You can visit an herbalist, a Chinese doctor, or other alternative healers with the stated and specific goal of getting pregnant. Acupuncture, in particular, has become a favorite of many lesbians. Inserting these small, thin needles into the skin is believed to help correct imbalances in the body that may be preventing pregnancy. An experienced alternative healer will be familiar with remedies and treatments for encouraging fertility and conception, and she may become a trusted ally along your path to pregnancy. You don't have to wait till you receive a diagnosis of infertility to seek out these treatments, either. Many women try these treatments concurrently with Western-oriented medical care for a more holistic approach to conception and pregnancy.

That Line in the Sand

The longer you try to get pregnant, the more desperate you are likely to feel. As time goes by, you may be more willing to take fertility drugs, for example. We all draw a line we're not willing to cross regarding medical intervention. Frequently, this line gets pushed farther and farther back as the periods keep coming and there's no baby in sight. This is normal, so don't beat yourself up about it. Even though my periods were regular, after six unsuccessful inseminations I, too, was considering fertility drugs. Thankfully, attempt number seven turned out to be the lucky one for me.

Fertility Drugs

There are several reasons why women may experience significant problems conceiving a child. One of the most common and most treatable causes is irregular periods—and therefore irregular ovulation. If women don't ovulate, they are said to be "anovulatory." Causes of this include glandular problems and certain types of hormonal imbalances. It can be really difficult to know when to inseminate when you're not able to pinpoint your ovulation. If you are not ovulating at all, there is no opportunity for an egg to be fertilized and for you to become pregnant.

By far the most popular way of coping with this is by taking the fertility drug clomiphene citrate. This drug is often referred to by one of its brand names, Clomid; its other brand name is Serophene. Clomid regulates ovulation by stimulating estrogen production. It is also used to treat polycystic ovary syndrome.

Clomid is taken orally, one 50 mg dose per day for five days, on your cycle's third through seventh days. This may be increased to 100mg as needed. Clomid has a high rate of success among women without significant fertility problems. About 80 percent of women using it ovulate, and about 40 percent go on to become pregnant within two or three cycles. In fact, some fertility doctors put you on Clomid right away, even if you are ovulating and have no history of infertility. They want to stack the odds in your favor, starting immediately, and Clomid is their first choice for doing so.

The average cost of one 50 mg dose of Clomid is about $10, so treatment costs about $50 per cycle. If it is going to work, it generally does so in the first month or two of use. Like most interventions, Clomid is not a miracle drug, and some physicians believe it is overprescribed. Clomid can dry up helpful cervical mucus (some women are given estrogen to prevent this) and may increase the risk of ovarian cancer later in life. It can make you feel moody and nauseated, blur your vision, and give you headaches. It also carries about a 10 percent risk for multiple births, because, according to Leland Traiman, director of Rainbow Flag Health Services, it can "kick more eggs out of your ovaries."

Sometimes Clomid is combined with the follicle-ripening drug Pergonal. Traiman calls Pergonal a "quantum leap above" Clomid in effectiveness. Pergonal is a gonadotropin (a hormone that stimulates the gonads) that works well with other assisted reproductive technologies. It is expensive, however, running $2,000 to $5,000 per cycle. It carries a risk as high as 40 percent for multiple births. Pergonal is injected for seven to 12 days; your partner can deliver the shots, if she cares to.

Other injectable fertility drugs include Fertinex, Repronex, and Follistim. It may surprise you to learn that some of these drugs, like Pergonal, are made from the urine of menopausal women! The job of all of these drugs is to dramatically increase the number of mature eggs that your body releases every month. You will have to get frequent transvaginal ultrasounds and blood tests to ensure that your body is coping with the hormones and maturing the eggs. Most women stay on these drugs for only a few cycles at a time. You may experience side effects including bloating and weight gain. And it's not unusual for these drugs to work too well—you could develop symptoms of ovarian hyperstimulation syndrome, caused by the rapid swelling of your ovaries. Talk about too much of a good thing!

> I was on Follistim and had successfully conceived with what I thought was going to be our second child. We had one son already, aged two, also conceived with fertility drugs. During my exam, the hospital fire alarm went off, so we couldn't hear what the doctor was saying to us about my ultrasound. So he pointed to the image and held up one finger for the first heartbeat he found, then another. Then he looked straight at us as he held up a third. Three heartbeats! We were so stunned we didn't know what to say. Finally, over the ringing of the bell, my partner sputtered out, "Does this mean we're having one of each?" It took us a while to really get that we were actually having triplets—three babies. I went on to have two boys, and a girl. One of each, indeed! —Deanna

Some women may have naturally low progesterone levels and cannot support a pregnancy even if sperm meets egg. They are said to have an "inadequate luteal phase," the luteal phase being the time after ovulation. These women may be prescribed extra progesterone via pills, suppositories, or injections of a drug such as Pergonal to keep them from menstruating. A new progesterone gel, which is absorbed directly into the uterus, can be inserted daily and has fewer side effects than injectable progesterone. With the boost of extra progesterone, any fertilized eggs have a chance to implant and not be miscarried. Although it may take some time before a woman suspects she has low progesterone, once diagnosed with a blood test she is often treated successfully.

Do remember that some fertility drugs including Pergonal (but usually not Clomid) can affect the results of ovulation predictor kits.

Multiple Births

A word about fertility drugs and multiple births. As more and more women use these drugs to become pregnant, the rate of multiple births continues to go up. The multiples produced by fertility drugs are said to be nonidentical because they are produced by different eggs fertilized by different sperm. That is, more eggs are made accessible for fertilization each month. The more eggs your body releases, the more can be fertilized by the sperm, and if several eggs implant, you will have several babies!

If you are doing IVF, usually several eggs are routinely fertilized. Thus, the odds are high that at least two of the batch will implant, and you will have twins or more.

Apart from the bond they undoubtedly share by being from multiple births, children who are born as nonidentical multiples are no more closely related than regular siblings—they just come all at once! But they are genetically different from identical twins, who have split from a single egg fertilized by a single sperm and thus share the same genetic material.

It is also possible that in a batch of triplets or quadruplets two children will be identical twins split from the same egg, while the other one or two are nonidentical. Some women are naturally prone to producing twins—a genetic tendency in some families that often skips a generation. So if your maternal grandmother was a twin, the odds are good that you will also produce twins.

The chance that you'll have to deal with giving birth to multiples when using fertility drugs is very real. Before you begin using such drugs, especially in the gonadotropin family, it's important that you understand their side effects and consider whether you're prepared to have twins, triplets, or even more children! Online bulletin boards that focus on fertility issues offer numerous comments about the side effects of various drugs; there are also bulletin boards for the mothers of multiples.

Selective reduction, whereby certain less viable fetuses in a group of multiples are aborted, is a topic of much discussion. Unfortunately, selective reduction can also lead to miscarriage of the entire pregnancy.

Selective reduction is not considered an issue for women carrying four or fewer fetuses, unless the health of one or more of the babies is in peril in utero.

Taking It One Step Further

I tried for a year to get pregnant at home with frozen sperm. Then I had three IUIs, again with no luck. After taking off a few months to chill out, I decided to just throw down all my money and try in vitro fertilization. The first time I tried it, I got pregnant. Drastic, maybe, but I got my baby! —Lois

Once you've realized that you're stuck, how do you make the decision to take your conception journey one step further? It will be an easy and obvious choice if you've got the driving desire and the resources to make it happen. Some coupled lesbians who have trouble getting pregnant try switching roles, with the other partner attempting pregnancy. Lesbians have been paving the way in yet another pregnancy path—taking one partner's fertilized eggs and placing them in her lover's uterus for gestation. This is known as ovum donation. In this way, both women are biologically related to the baby. It is still relatively rare in the community, but it is happening. If you are contemplating ovum donation for your partner, make sure that you carefully discuss and document your legal rights to the child, and don't waive parental rights lightly.

There are a couple of other options, besides egg donation and increasingly potent injectable drugs, for those with the money, the time, and the willpower to attempt them. One of these is gamete intrafallopian transfer, in which a woman's mature eggs are taken from the ovaries and placed with the sperm in the fallopian tubes, where it is hoped the two shall meet. Another is in vitro fertilization. If you are over 40 and have already tried several times to become pregnant, or remain pregnant, in vitro may be for you. It is tremendously expensive, often around $12,000 to $20,000 per attempt, but your insurance may cover most of it. Also, you must take expensive drugs for egg retrieval that can cause serious side effects; the procedures involved are not pleasant. Nevertheless, in vitro is becoming more common among lesbians determined to have children.

While some women have luck with these procedures, for others, they are simply another expensive round of frustration and side effects.

What Some Women Have to Say About Clomiphene and Other Fertility Drugs

Don't be afraid of fertility drugs. Just because we're lesbians doesn't mean that we have to do everything naturally, and it can waste a lot of time. I waited through nine months of inseminations before wondering whether I ought to ask about fertility drugs. Now looking back at my two pregnancies, I realize there's no way I would have gotten pregnant either time without Clomid. And lookie at what I got for it! —Maria

When we started trying to conceive, my partner was on Clomid because of a history of irregular ovulation. After six months of trying at home (frozen sperm, two inseminations per month) we decided we needed some help. We were referred to a reproductive endocrinologist, who kept my partner on Clomid and added Metrodin (to stimulate egg production) and hCG, to help launch the eggs. The first time we tried this combo we got pregnant! Needless to say, we are very thankful to Western medicine for the help we got in having our twin boys. —Gwyneth

I'm 40, with no known health or reproductive problems. I'm on progesterone, 200 mg 2x a day. During my last cycle I used a hCG shot and then inseminated 36 hours later. Happily, I got pregnant. Unfortunately, the pregnancy didn't last. Despite the warnings, I had no side effects from the hCG shot. In fact even the shot didn't really hurt. I was kind of amazed —Juliette

Most lesbians don't investigate these options, given their high cost and the decreased emphasis many of us place on the importance of carrying on our own genetic line. When we bump up against the bigger walls, many consider options like adoption instead. But you should consult a fertility expert for more information on these treatments.

It is possible that structural problems with the uterus or cervix prevent you from becoming pregnant. Such problems are common among "DES

I had a low progesterone level, which was picked up very early in the process by my fertility specialist. I had to bump up the level of Clomid to 150 mg before it raised my progesterone enough to be at a normal level. Two tries at a normal level and we were pregnant. —Katriana

I just had my first IUI last week after an injection of Pregnyl. The shot made me feel terrible, very achy and exhausted and dizzy. But I'm willing to go through this again if it helps me get pregnant. —Roanne

My regular ob/gyn doesn't do inseminations in her office, so we decided to try using a fertility doctor. First thing he did was check my progesterone level, saw that it was too low, and put me on Clomid. I could have tried getting pregnant for a whole year before we realized it wouldn't happen. What a nightmare that would have been! I was pregnant three months later. —Leesa

I took Clomid in combination with Repronex injections. I have heard that women have hugely varied reactions to the drugs, from depression to elation, but I was symptom-free. —Anya

I took 50 mg of Clomid for two months and got pregnant on the second try. I went to a fertility specialist and he used an ultrasound to check for viable eggs, then I was inseminated by IUI. The only thing I didn't like about the drug was that it caused me lots of cramping. But it was worth it! —Stephanie

daughters." DES (diethylstilbestrol) was given erroneously to women from the 1940s through the early 1970s to prevent miscarriage. Unfortunately, due to exposure in the womb, many of the children subsequently born were deformed or infertile. If you ascertain you are a DES daughter, you should consult a specialist before you begin trying to get pregnant.

Frustratingly, some fertility problems are impossible to diagnose. Certain women just cannot get pregnant, no matter what they try. I know a bisexual woman who has had every health test recommended, tried every fertility drug available, and even slept with two different men, all to no avail. She was pronounced in perfect health time after time, but she could never conceive. She still has no idea why.

Miscarriage and Mourning

My first pregnancy ended at about three weeks. I'm sure I noticed only because we knew I was pregnant and were paying such close attention. I had been feeling unwell and then got a period that was heavy, clumpy, and just not normal. I know that feeling as sick as I did, and the pregnancy ending as it did, meant that all was not well, and it was probably for the best that this happened. However, it's been several years and I still wonder and mourn about what might have been. Three months after this loss, I got pregnant again and had a healthy pregnancy and delivery. —Francesca

We had a miscarriage at about ten weeks into our first pregnancy. It is a grieving process like any other. Allow yourselves time to heal and hold each other close. It is such a hard time, but having this experience does at least show you can get pregnant. Keep the faith and ask your doctor if there is anything that you could do next time to increase your success, like progesterone suppositories.
—Audre

After a very sad miscarriage, Sally was told she had diabetes. It took us a year and a half and a lot of learning to get her blood sugar under control so we could get pregnant again. —Carla

Statistics show that most women who suffer miscarriage go on to have a healthy pregnancy later. While there can be circumstances that clearly indicate a serious health problem in the mother, often there is nothing really wrong, and the miscarriage is no one's fault. Nature has her ways of dealing with imperfect fetuses, and the most common is to flush them out of the mother's body before they become viable. It's estimated that as many as one-third of all pregnancies end in an early miscarriage before the first 20 weeks. (This number is high because it includes pregnancies that end as early as a few weeks.)

If you were not tracking your cycles or trying so hard to conceive, you may not even notice an early miscarriage. It may manifest itself as a heavy period, or you may experience cramping and clotting. Some women claim they knew they miscarried even before they took a pregnancy test, because they had such a difficult, late period. While nothing can be done to stop an early miscarriage once it is occurring, steps can be taken to prevent them in the future. In some cases, intervention to halt a miscarriage in later pregnancy can be taken as a pregnancy progresses. In any case, call a doctor immediately if you suspect anything is wrong or you experience any bleeding or cramps at any time after a positive pregnancy test.

Women older than 35 may have more miscarriages, but it can happen to women of any age. Because miscarriage can be a sign of diseases such as chlamydia, rubella, and lupus, you should always get a checkup after a miscarriage and before attempting pregnancy again. Healing emotionally and physically from a miscarriage, like any loss, takes time. You will need to grieve a bit before you move on, whether your pregnancy was just a few weeks along, or, heartbreakingly, close to term. Balance your need to take this time against your clicking biological clock. Find support for your loss in empathetic friends, books, and online support groups.

Coming to the Fork in the Road

Don't forget about all the women who've gone through extreme measures and many years in their journey to pregnancy. I've tried home insemination, IUIs, fresh sperm, frozen sperm, Clomid, Pergonal, in vitro treatments, acupuncture, hypnosis, and a lot of therapy! As lesbians it's difficult enough to find support for what I consider a natural part of being a woman. But I found that the most devastating thing about infertility is the guilt and shame associated with it and the lack of support, particularly in the lesbian community. —Jess

It's a sad fact that not every woman who wants a baby can have one biologically. While women younger than 35 often have better luck, infertility can be any woman's problem. However, if you've waited till your forties to start this journey, it may be a rough one. A prolonged period of trying to conceive, or multiple miscarriages, may mean your body is trying to tell you it is too late. Eggs harden and age, and by your mid-forties, the fact is, most are simply no longer viable.

At some point, we may reach a fork in the road on our journey to parenthood. In one direction lies the road to biological motherhood: what we have lusted for and spent some years and thousands of dollars trying to achieve. But in the other direction another, equally open, road beckons. It may be heartbreaking initially to give up the biological path, but once you do, another world will open up to you. As Helen Keller wrote, "When one door of happiness closes, another opens, but often we look so long at the closed door that we do not see the one which has been opened for us."

There are many ways other than biological motherhood to bring children into your life: mentoring, fostering, coparenting, surrogacy, adoption. (Of course, you can explore all these options even if you're fertile.)

Most states welcome lesbian foster and adoptive parents. You may be especially welcome if you are interested in foster parenting or are willing to adopt a special-needs child. Unfortunately, other states have archaic and homophobic laws barring gay people from providing a home to children in need. There are ways around the system, including having one partner adopt as a "single" parent. A large number of agencies handling both domestic and international adoptions welcome lesbian couples and single lesbian mothers. However, the laws regarding which countries allow international adoption by "single" women in North America continually change, so don't count on adoption from a particular country until you have the current facts. Word of mouth from other adoptive families and some Internet research will lead you to companies that currently deal with lesbians and the countries that accept such adoptions.

Finally, if you decide that you have come to the end of your own path to parenthood, know that there will always be children around you to love. You can volunteer at schools or libraries, or become a Big Sister, a "respite" foster parent, or even a favorite auntie to a friend with children. It is not the same as giving birth or having your own child. But what a gift you will be able to give to children already around you in your world.

Chapter

7

So You're Finally Pregnant! Welcome to the World of Eating, Sleeping, and Puking

Think you're pregnant? Or just want to believe you are? Read on for everything you'll need to know.

Is It Pregnancy—or Just PMS?

If you're like most lesbians trying to get pregnant, immediately after insemination you will begin thinking you notice signs of pregnancy. This contrasts with women whose pregnancies are unplanned, many of whom might not even get a clue till they miss a period (or two!) and subsequently upchuck in the toilet. Of course, because lesbians have to be so methodical about all this, and it's costing some of us a fortune besides, we'll be the ones counting the hours till our period is one minute late!

Since most pregnancy books are written for straight women, the books usually assume you've already missed a period before they fill you in on a bare minimum of symptoms. But here we can acknowledge the truth: if you've never been a hypochondriac by nature, you will become one when you start trying to conceive. You'll fully believe (and rightly so) that every possible little symptom *may be a sign* of pregnancy. So let's just get a few facts out of the way.

How Do You Know You're Pregnant?

Some women claim to know, the minute they inseminate, if it has taken. Others want to believe this but are proven wrong when their period blood comes. The truth is probably that when we're hoping we're pregnant, every possible sign becomes greatly magnified. It doesn't help to know that the very early signs of pregnancy are exactly like the symptoms of PMS. In fact, the month I actually got pregnant, I was convinced I couldn't be, because I had such bad PMS-type symptoms. I thought I was going to bleed any minute, and I refused to break down and take a pregnancy test till day 34 of my usually 28-to-30-day cycle.

Very Early Signs of Pregnancy

Focusing on the earliest signs of pregnancy, here are some things to look for. Some women experience these symptoms as early as a few days after insemination.

- Your breasts become sore
- You notice a heightened sense of smell
- You begin feeling slightly nauseated
- You see a slight amount of spotting around the time of your period (due to implantation of the egg)
- You feel tired and emotionally vulnerable

Much like PMS, no? So how do you tell the difference? You really can't, unless something obvious happens, such as throwing up. And let's hope you have as little of *that* as possible!

Taking a Pregnancy Test

Most pregnancy tests work by testing for a hormone called hCG (human chorionic gonadotropin), which is produced by your tiny embryo and begins appearing in your urine as early as a week after conception. It builds up quickly until the time it is reliably detectable, which is the first day of your missed period. This is also about when the fertilized egg implants itself in the uterine wall. Although home pregnancy tests are becoming ever more sensitive, if you do a test before the first day of your missed period you may get a false negative. So save your money and wait till that day or later to take the test!

Pregnancy tests are easy to use. You simply hold one end of a stick under your morning urine stream as you pee into the toilet, or collect some urine in a clean jar and dip the test stick in it. Then you set the strip down on a flat dry surface as you wait for the result. The result appears in a window next to a control line that is usually purple or another color. If you are pregnant, a test line matching the control line quickly appears. If no line appears, you have tested too early, or you are not pregnant. Even if the test line comes up very faintly, you are pregnant. There is no such thing as being "a little bit pregnant." The test looks for hCG. If it finds it in your system, you are pregnant.

Tests are also available now that work the same way but display the words "Pregnant" or "Not Pregnant" instead of a test line. This should help resolve any question women feel when they look at their test results!

Some women leave the room while they wait for their test result. Not me! I sat there and watched as that second line came up so fast and strong that all I could do was stare at it and say "Oh my God, oh my God" over and over again. The elation I felt at that moment was overwhelming. It was the most surreal and happy moment of my life.

Many women actually do not believe a positive pregnancy test result. It is almost too much to believe that after trying so hard to make it happen, it has. To make it even harder to believe, when you look in the mirror you appear the same as you did five minutes ago, before you knew you were pregnant. Make sure you have a second test available, as you will likely want to test again. No doubt that second test will, unbelievably, again tell you that you're pregnant! After doing my first test I had to run to the drugstore and buy another—I simply couldn't believe I was pregnant.

If your results give you the good news that you're pregnant, let me be the first to offer congratulations on this momentous occasion. You've done it!

You Know—but Should You Tell?

After all your planning and trying and hoping, it may be tempting to want to tell everyone your happy news right away. I know I could barely restrain myself from shouting, "I'm pregnant!" at the top of my lungs as I walked down the street in my neighborhood. Because as lesbians we're actively trying to get pregnant, we tend to find out very early if we're pregnant or not—often we know on the first day of our missed period. But while you may want to tell everyone right away, there are a

What's Happening in There?

Weeks 1–2 You aren't even pregnant yet, but these first two weeks of your menstrual cycle count as the beginning of your pregnancy. That's why, technically, you'll be 40 weeks pregnant—a whopping ten months—when your baby arrives. Now is when the body prepares for the possibility of pregnancy, with the eggs ripening in fluid-filled sacs called follicles.

Week 3 This is the magic week! Ovulation occurs when the ripened ovum is swept into the fallopian tube, and if you're going to become pregnant, it will be penetrated by one sperm, with the help of others trying. The egg accepts that sperm and immediately closes itself to the others. The fertilized egg then begins to divide, floating down the fallopian tube toward the uterus. It is now called a zygote.

Weeks 4–5 This is the time you will probably miss a period and suspect you could be pregnant. Of course, if you are like most lesbians trying to get pregnant, you have already stocked up on pregnancy tests! The zygote (now a ball of cells) has implanted in the wall of the uterus, and a placenta is starting to grow. The embryo is about a quarter inch long.

---

few reasons to wait. The main one is that most miscarriages happen very early on in a pregnancy, often before most women are even aware they're pregnant.

An early miscarriage may take the form of a very heavy, late period, so if you didn't know you were pregnant, you might not even notice. Every woman who miscarries finds it a painful experience, but women who have shared their pregnancy news early on only to miscarry find it even more unbearable. For not only have their hopes for pregnancy been dashed, they must also tell everyone they lost the baby. Further, they may

Weeks 6–8 The embryo has a beating heart but is still less than an inch long, about the size of a large bean or a berry. It has small arms and the beginning of toes, ears, eyelids, mouth, and intestines. The amniotic sac has begun to form. The neural tube, the very important precursor to the brain, spinal cord, and nervous system, is forming. Make sure you're taking your prenatal vitamins to get enough folic acid.

Weeks 9–10 Your baby is now an inch-long fetus that moves, has actual facial features, and hands and feet with toes, and almost looks like a teeny, tiny human being. Its rudimentary nervous system is working, and many of its organs are beginning to function. Because of this, toxins like cigarette smoke and alcohol are especially harmful to your fetus in the first trimester.

Weeks 11–12 Your baby is growing rapidly as you approach the end of your first trimester. It should be close to three inches long now and weigh up to several ounces. It has a beating heart and a developing umbilical cord, which are about to begin circulating blood between the fetus and the placenta. It is a fully formed miniature human being. By the end of your first trimester you will most likely be able to hear the whoosh of its heartbeat with the aid of a device called a Doppler. You can't feel it yet, but the baby is already moving around and kicking inside you.

have to deal with constant questions like "So, how's the baby?" from people who don't yet know of the loss.

However, often the news is just so exciting, particularly if you've finally been successful after a long period of trying, that you'll want to tell people, selectively, right from the start. Usually women tell their partner first, and then perhaps a select circle of good friends and close family members. Then the news will start spreading, so you may want to actively plan who finds out, and when. Otherwise, there may be some hurt feelings if certain people don't hear the word directly from you!

How Will People React?

When I told my mother I was finally pregnant after months of try-ing, her first reaction was, "Are you sure that's what you want?" I was really hurt, because it seemed like she was saying it was only a mistake! She never asked my straight brother that, and their son was unplanned! —Mimi

My mother was cautious about my partner and me having a baby. She especially didn't understand how the baby fit into her world, since it was my wife who had him. But once she saw the baby, all misgivings were behind her. You should hear her sweet-talk the baby now! He's the light of her life! —Brenda

The reaction many of us worry about most is from our parents. It's true that for some parents this is the best news you could ever deliver, and they'll share your joy right from moment one. If you don't have living parents, it may be sad not to be able to share news of an upcoming grandchild with them. If you're estranged from your family, as some gay people are, you may decide to wait to tell them. Or, the news may bring you closer. The fact is, it probably will. Even if they don't like your lifestyle or your partner, or don't approve of your being a single parent, once they see their grandchild, they'll probably fall in love. It may be hard for some parents initially to accept a grandchild as theirs if it is a child your part-ner, not you, has borne. But time has a way of healing, and if they see that you are a dedicated parent to the child, and very much a part of a family unit, they'll probably come around eventually.

It may also help to tell your birth family, or your partner's, about legal protections you have arranged for your partner and child, such as a sec-ond-parent adoption. Just having a will or a parenting agreement pre-pared by a lawyer shows your intent. Your parents may not get exactly what a "second parent" adoption is, but everyone understands and respects the finality and responsibilities of adoption. And most people take legal documents quite seriously. So if are looking for further proof to present to your biological family about what your partner and child mean to you, and what you mean to one another, use the legal system to your advantage wherever possible. As we've previously discussed in this book, seeing a competent attorney in your state *before* you begin trying to conceive is a good first step.

Certainly, telling supportive friends your good news will be the easy part. But how will more casual acquaintances react? Many lesbians do not understand why some dykes want to become mothers. They may give you a hard time about it, or ask offensive or invasive questions about your methods of conceiving, your pregnancy, or your ability to parent a child. Remember, you do not have to answer any question that makes you uncomfortable, or defend your right to have a child, to anyone— even other lesbians! With work colleagues and other straight folks in the general population, you may experience more curiosity than overt homophobia, depending on where you live. Some people still can't hide their distaste at the idea of bringing children up in a gay household. But remember that you will be setting the example here. Showing your happiness and your preparedness to be a good mother will go farther than any argument about the appropriateness of your family. And as more and more lesbians have children, and lesbian families appear to be truly everywhere, prejudice will be chipped away.

When Are You Due?

Based on the medical model of 28-day cycles, your estimated date of delivery is 266 days from the date of conception, or 280 days from the first day of your last period. The chart shown on page 118 makes it easy to find your estimated due date, based on the first day of your last missed period. To use the chart, locate the month and day of that first day of bleeding, then, in the line below, look at the second month and the date. That is your estimated due date.

Note that, according to medical standards, by the first day of your missed period (the date many women start testing for pregnancy), you are already considered several weeks pregnant! This timetable equates to 40 weeks from the start of your last menstrual period—more like ten months of pregnancy than the expected nine! Because every woman's cycle length is different, keep in mind that your estimated due date is just that—an estimate. A healthy pregnancy can last anywhere between 38 and 42 weeks, and only about 5 percent of babies are actually born on their due dates. First-time moms are usually a bit late. Still, a due date gives us something to strive for; a marker of how far we have to go. It will help us measure the passage of time along the way, and help us understand the important milestones on this amazing journey. This becomes

Your Due Date

January	1 2 3 4 5 6 7 8 9 10 11 12 13 14 15 16 17 18 19 20 21 22 23 24 25 26 27 28 29 30 31
Oct. / Nov.	8 9 10 11 12 13 14 15 16 17 18 19 20 21 22 23 24 25 26 27 28 29 30 31 1 2 3 4 5 6 7
February	1 2 3 4 5 6 7 8 9 10 11 12 13 14 15 16 17 18 19 20 21 22 23 24 25 26 27 28
Nov. / Dec.	8 9 10 11 12 13 14 15 16 17 18 19 20 21 22 23 24 25 26 27 28 29 30 1 2 3 4 5
March	1 2 3 4 5 6 7 8 9 10 11 12 13 14 15 16 17 18 19 20 21 22 23 24 25 26 27 28 29 30 31
Dec. / Jan.	6 7 8 9 10 11 12 13 14 15 16 17 18 19 20 21 22 23 24 25 26 27 28 29 30 31 1 2 3 4 5
April	1 2 3 4 5 6 7 8 9 10 11 12 13 14 15 16 17 18 19 20 21 22 23 24 25 26 27 28 29 30
Jan. / Feb.	6 7 8 9 10 11 12 13 14 15 16 17 18 19 20 21 22 23 24 25 26 27 28 29 30 31 1 2 3 4
May	1 2 3 4 5 6 7 8 9 10 11 12 13 14 15 16 17 18 19 20 21 22 23 24 25 26 27 28 29 30 31
Feb. / March	5 6 7 8 9 10 11 12 13 14 15 16 17 18 19 20 21 22 23 24 25 26 27 28 1 2 3 4 5 6 7
June	1 2 3 4 5 6 7 8 9 10 11 12 13 14 15 16 17 18 19 20 21 22 23 24 25 26 27 28 29 30
March / April	8 9 10 11 12 13 14 15 16 17 18 19 20 21 22 23 24 25 26 27 28 29 30 31 1 2 3 4 5 6
July	1 2 3 4 5 6 7 8 9 10 11 12 13 14 15 16 17 18 19 20 21 22 23 24 25 26 27 28 29 30 31
April / May	7 8 9 10 11 12 13 14 15 16 17 18 19 20 21 22 23 24 25 26 27 28 29 30 1 2 3 4 5 6 7
August	1 2 3 4 5 6 7 8 9 10 11 12 13 14 15 16 17 18 19 20 21 22 23 24 25 26 27 28 29 30 31
May / June	8 9 10 11 12 13 14 15 16 17 18 19 20 21 22 23 24 25 26 27 28 29 30 31 1 2 3 4 5 6 7
September	1 2 3 4 5 6 7 8 9 10 11 12 13 14 15 16 17 18 19 20 21 22 23 24 25 26 27 28 29 30
June / July	8 9 10 11 12 13 14 15 16 17 18 19 20 21 22 23 24 25 26 27 28 29 30 1 2 3 4 5 6 7
October	1 2 3 4 5 6 7 8 9 10 11 12 13 14 15 16 17 18 19 20 21 22 23 24 25 26 27 28 29 30 31
July / Aug.	8 9 10 11 12 13 14 15 16 17 18 19 20 21 22 23 24 25 26 27 28 29 30 31 1 2 3 4 5 6 7
November	1 2 3 4 5 6 7 8 9 10 11 12 13 14 15 16 17 18 19 20 21 22 23 24 25 26 27 28 29 30
Aug. / Sept.	8 9 10 11 12 13 14 15 16 17 18 19 20 21 22 23 24 25 26 27 28 29 30 31 1 2 3 4 5 6
December	1 2 3 4 5 6 7 8 9 10 11 12 13 14 15 16 17 18 19 20 21 22 23 24 25 26 27 28 29 30 31
Sept. / Oct.	7 8 9 10 11 12 13 14 15 16 17 18 19 20 21 22 23 24 25 26 27 28 29 30 1 2 3 4 5 6 7

especially important in medical checkups. "When are you due?" will be the question most often asked about your pregnancy, so get used to giving out this bit of information.

Medical Tests You Can Expect Now

After you've confirmed with a home pregnancy kit that you're pregnant, you'll probably have a nice, long visit with your nurse-practitioner or doctor. Possibly you'll be given an "official" pregnancy test, using either your blood or your urine. You may choose to waive this, if, like me, you took multiple home pregnancy tests. If you haven't been seeing an RE regularly, and have been inseminating at home or through a sperm bank, you'll be given a general physical exam including a breast exam, a pelvic exam (to check for infections as well as the size and position of your ovaries and uterus), and a Pap smear. On your first medical visit as a pregnant woman, you will probably get other tests as well: blood pressure and urinalysis (expect these at every visit hereafter); a blood test to determine blood type, Rh type, and exposure to rubella and toxoplasmosis; and most likely tests for STIs and HIV. You will be weighed, and you may be offered an early sonogram if you have previously miscarried.

If you see a doctor for any other reason during your first trimester, it is imperative that you mention to the doctor that you are pregnant, no matter what you are being treated for. Now is also the time to lay off any pain medications you routinely take, such as ibuprofen, which can be extremely harmful to the developing fetus. Talk to your doctor about how you can manage any chronic pain or illness you have in ways that will be safe for your baby.

Sonogram, or Ultrasound

Ultrasounds have become rather routine in prenatal care, but it is still up to you to decide if you want them. In fact, the American College of

Obstetricians and Gynecologists questions the use of "routine" ultrasound. You don't have to agree to an ultrasound, or any other prenatal test that you don't want. You can choose to forgo ultrasounds early in your pregnancy. In fact, midwives often recommend postponing any medical intervention for the first few weeks, and instead rely on blood tests to check in with the baby.

Most women choose to have at least one ultrasound. If you've taken fertility drugs or undergone IVF, you may have received several ultrasounds by the time your pregnancy is even a few weeks along. If you've conceived without IVF or fertility drugs, your first ultrasound will likely be given some time between the sixteenth and twentieth weeks. If you have previously miscarried, you may be offered one earlier. If you're feeling anxious because of past losses, an early ultrasound can be very reassuring by showing you that the tiny fetus is developing normally.

In an ultrasound, high-pitched sonar sound waves are reflected off your organs, creating an image on a TV-like screen. The technician looks for the location of the placenta and signs of the health of your growing baby—as well as how many babies are actually in there! Ultrasounds are also used to determine how far along you are in your pregnancy, but if you've conceived through insemination, you generally know to the day when this happened.

The usual procedure for an ultrasound is for you to enter a special room, pull up your shirt, lie on a table, and have your belly smeared with gooey gel. Then the technician presses down on your belly with a hand-held device called a transducer, and the image is transmitted to the screen. It's exciting to see the image of your baby for the first time, even if it does look like an alien! I suggest bringing your partner or a good friend with you to share this moment. It's one of the big ones! Usually you will get a Polaroid-type picture or two of the baby to take home with you. I kept one for my daughter's baby book. Depending on the hospital, you can sometimes order better pictures or even a short videotape copy of this ultrasound footage.

Some people disparage ultrasounds because they feel the test doesn't provide enough useful information and may disturb the baby. While I certainly don't advise taking any unnecessary tests, it can be very reassuring not only to hear that everything is fine but actually to see a photo of your baby. Some women also find out the sex of their baby during their first ultrasound, but generally, if the test is performed before 20 weeks, you are not able to tell yet. Keep in mind, too, that what a technician sees is open to interpretation—you may be told you're having the opposite of what's actually in there!

While there should be no pain associated with an ultrasound, I found drinking the suggested amount of water beforehand very uncomfortable. I also felt, intuitively, that my baby did not like this sonar invasion, and I opted not to have another scan for the rest of my pregnancy.

Changes During the First Trimester

Here Come the Real Changes!

Hormones are now surging through your body, and the changes you are undergoing, even this early in your pregnancy, are monumental. Your heart is working harder, your blood volume is increasing, your breasts are growing in preparation for feeding the baby, your uterus is enlarging and moving, and your baby's neurological systems are forming. Let's have a look at some of the things you may be going through now.

Morning Sickness

It's almost impossible to describe morning sickness to someone who hasn't experienced it. But I'll try. Imagine the worst hangover of your life, complete with the urge to throw up and an overwhelming sense of fatigue thrown in for good measure. Now imagine feeling that way for three or four months. That's about how it feels to have a bad case of morning sickness. Except it's not just in the morning—it's all day long, with the nausea often peaking first thing in the morning and again later in the day, either in the evening or in the middle of the night. In addition to plain old nausea, it often felt as though someone had their hands around my neck and was squeezing just hard enough to make me want to be sick. Very unpleasant!

What makes pregnant women so nauseated? Part of it is hormones, and part of it is the tremendous changes taking place in your body. These include coping with surging hormones, extra nutritional needs, a shifting metabolism, and the extra bile that is likely to collect in your stomach. When your tummy is empty (as it is first thing in the morning), the sick feeling can be intensely awful.

Every woman's experience is different, and some women never even get morning sickness. There is no way to predict how bad your morning sickness will be, and a second or third pregnancy will often result in a completely different experience than your first.

However, morning sickness is not all bad. Studies prove that women who have had morning sickness go on to have mostly normal pregnancies and actually suffer fewer miscarriages than women who never get it. So chin up! You may think you'll never get through the next few months, but somehow you will.

Tricks to Combat Morning Sickness

There are a number of tactics you can employ to combat morning sickness. Here are a few that have worked both for me and for other women I know.

KEEP YOUR STOMACH FULL
Many women find that avoiding an empty tummy is a good way to keep from feeling sick at any time of day—or night. This is where the old cracker remedy comes in. It's believed that munching on crackers, particularly in the night or early-morning hours, keeps the nausea at bay. This is probably true, since crackers, or plain bread, soak up the bile and fill the stomach quickly. Personally, I can't stand crackers, and the thought of eating them when I was already feeling sick was completely unappealing. What worked much better for me was to keep an apple by my bedside, and every time I'd wake up during the night to pee I'd just take a bite out of the apple. Really tart ones like Granny Smiths seemed to be the most comforting. During the day, sucking on sour candy also seemed to do the trick. Try a Preggie Pop made especially for morning sickness (order from www.threelollies.com). And that old standby ginger ale lived up to its reputation as a stomach settler. Since most commercial ginger ales don't actually contain real ginger, look for health-food sodas that list ginger as an ingredient. Ginger tea can help, too. Sucking on a lemon when the nausea hits is a remedy many women swear by.

USE PAPER PLATES
True, this is wasteful. But in my first few months of pregnancy the thought of cooking food was so repulsive that I almost couldn't bear to be in my kitchen. And the sight of a dirty plate could make me retch. So a friend bought me a huge stack of paper plates, and this enabled me to eat in my own house again. Pots and pans, of course, were another matter. Thank heavens for take-out food!

GET SOME AIR

Your house (and of course, everywhere else you go, too) may suddenly smell terrible to you. Burn scented candles at home if this helps. Avoid stinky places. Keep your house clean. Open your windows wide, letting the fresh air come streaming in. This can cut down on accumulated cooking odors and even low-level toxins in your home air. Get out of the house for a while. A walk around the block will get fresh air in your lungs and your body moving, healthy on all counts.

KEEP THE LITTER BOX CLEAN

I always keep the cat's litter box in my house very clean. Yet, nothing smelled as awful to me during my pregnancy. Because I had the super-sensitive nose of pregnancy, I had to hold my breath while changing it, then rush out of the room afterward to gulp fresh air. Many times, just looking at the box, even when it was clean, would make me gag. As we've already discussed, cat poop is not the healthiest thing for pregnant women to begin with (as I'm sure my body was trying to tell me), so be sure to wear rubber gloves every time you change the box.

TRY NOT TO TRIGGER YOUR GAG REFLEX

Even putting my toothbrush in my mouth was too much for me, some mornings, and I threw up a few times attempting to brush my teeth. But I didn't want to pass up brushing, because of the increased risk of gum disease for pregnant women. So, a few times, I simply used mouthwash and brushed for about five seconds. Use disposable toothbrushes or even just your finger, if you're really on the edge. By the same token, skip the prenatal vitamins when you feel you absolutely can't swallow one. Better to keep your breakfast down than just have a vitamin in your tummy.

KEEP EMERGENCY PROVISIONS WITH YOU

I felt like a freak carrying around ginger ale and Wild Berry Lifesavers everywhere I went for a few weeks, but it was a technique that worked for me. One possible cause of nausea is an overproduction of nasty thick saliva, and sucking on candy seems to thin it down. The ginger ale helped settle my stomach and made me burp up gas. Armed with both, I could face the world—barely! Through trial and error, you'll learn what works for you.

SNACK AT BEDTIME

A healthy snack at bedtime is almost always necessary to make sure the baby has nighttime nutrients. If you haven't eaten anything, the baby will just drain off your nutrients and make you feel sicker when you awaken. Keep nutritious snacks by your bed for middle-of-the-night noshing, and have high-protein foods like leftover cold chicken at the ready in the fridge.

TRUST YOUR INSTINCTS

If something doesn't appeal to you, foodwise, don't attempt to eat it. Listen to your body. Some people think morning sickness exists to keep women from eating things that are toxic or just no good for them during pregnancy. Whether you want to believe that or not, if your body says, "Come near me with that fish fillet and I'll upchuck," it may be best to eat the beef or tofu instead.

TRY ALTERNATIVE HEALING

Herbs and homeopathy may be helpful for nausea. I had good luck with taking the homeopathic drug Ipecacuanha (9c, though some recommend 30c) when my morning sickness was at its worst. I also took Pulsatilla (200ck) when I became overwrought emotionally. However, before you take any herbs or drugs, talk to an herbalist or homeopath (or your midwife or doctor). Read the *Wise Woman Herbal for the Childbearing Year*, by Susun Weed, for more ideas on this topic. Acupressure wristbands which press the nai-kan points in the wrists help some women. Acupuncture can also be helpful for morning sickness or other discomforts of pregnancy.

DRINK ENOUGH FLUIDS

Vomiting can easily dehydrate you. Drinking as much clear fluid as you can—especially water—is good for your body and for your baby.

DON'T GET TOO TIRED

Exhaustion makes morning sickness worse. Slow down! Accept help, and don't wear yourself out. Many pregnant women find they have to start taking more time off from their jobs—and their friends, lovers, and social engagements. Your body needs to rest and grow the baby. If you don't slow down on your own, you'll get sicker till you have to. Why let it get to that point?

If Symptoms Persist

Most women find morning sickness goes away sometime between the twelfth and eighteenth weeks. If the symptoms are more than you can bear, or you're starting to lose weight, it's important to see your doctor or midwife about this. You may be suffering from a severe form of morning sickness termed hyperemesis gravidarum. And you will need some help in dealing with this. If you don't get help, you may find yourself dehydrated and extremely sleep-deprived, and in the worst-case scenario, you will need to be given intravenous fluids in a hospital. As a last-ditch effort to curb acute nausea, you may be prescribed medication.

For a more detailed account of morning sickness, and the various theories and remedies associated with it, read *Managing Morning Sickness: A Survival Guide for Pregnant Women,* by Miriam Erick.

The Need to Feed

Newly pregnant women often develop a tremendous appetite. This is what happened to me: I just couldn't seem to get enough to eat. I would devour a huge meal and then be able to eat another just an hour later. It was quite astonishing! In part, this was because I found eating alleviated my all-day morning sickness. And I was just plain more hungry than I had ever been in my life. Since I'm not prone to overeat generally, I just listened to my body and ate what it seemed to want. Make sure you eat enough protein, and try to eat more frequent, smaller meals throughout the day if you never seem full. This will help keep your blood sugar level.

Food Cravings

Every pregnant woman seems to crave different things. The myth adage about pickles held some truth for me. I found the sourness of a good dill pickle a perfect cure for nausea. Pickles also provide sodium, which many pregnant women need. What I loved even more while pregnant was anything orange-colored—fresh oranges, orange popsicles, apricots, apricot nectar, tomatoes, tomato soup, and cantaloupe, as well as more unhealthy orange things like peach ring candies and canned Chef Boyardee Spaghetti and Meatballs. I can only deduce that this craving was due in part to my body's need for folic acid, which many orange foods have in abundance.

As my pregnancy progressed, and I learned how to eat better for my pregnant self, I started enjoying a wider variety of things, including salad, milk, and cold barbecued chicken. I continued to devour fruit, though, and have since learned that many women crave fruit while pregnant. If you have a partner, and even other children, involve the whole family in "eating well for baby." Rid the house of junk food and sodas, stock up on healthy snacks, and have lots of bottled water around. It's a great opportunity to all get healthier together.

Some Strange Symptoms of the First Trimester

POLICE-DOG NOSE

Most pregnant women develop a supersensitive sniffer. It's probably your body's way of detecting rotten or toxic foods, and you should always pay heed to Mother Nature's signals. Certain smells will probably make you want to heave after just one whiff. If these are food smells, don't eat those foods. If they're environmental, try to get rid of them or at least avoid them for a few months. For me it was Christmas trees, gasoline, raw fish, the cat's litter box, and anything cooking in my house. Tell your coworkers to stay out of your office if they reek of cologne, open a window if possible, and ensure that communal coffee pots in an office suite are shut off before the overcooked coffee smell turns rancid. My own mom said she knew she was pregnant with me when the smell of coffee made her throw up. A friend told me coffee "literally smelled like shit" to her while pregnant. Think all these triggers add up to a message? Yes, indeed, coffee is truly one of those things a pregnant gal should do without. Luckily, the worst aspects of this extreme sensitivity to smell will recede along with your morning sickness.

ATOMIC TITTIES

Forget PMS-type sore breasts. Soon you may experience the growth of what I term Atomic Titties. This means that not only will your breasts start growing, they will hurt like hell. I could barely stand the pain, and the thought of anyone else touching them, even gently, made me recoil in horror. This pain will subside sometime during your second trimester, but your breasts will stay large. They are preparing for the work of breast-feeding later on and will soon stop aching. Whether they will ever go back to your previous, smaller size is an altogether different question. Some women claim they keep their larger breasts after childbirth, but others find, as I did, that their breasts shrink to close their original size, even after nursing.

FAINTING

You can avoid fainting by making sure your blood-sugar level stays constant, getting up slowly from a seated position, and not getting over-tired. The one time I fainted was in my first trimester, when I forgot to eat an early-morning snack before heading out for breakfast with my girl-friend. We were in the restaurant, waiting for our food, when I felt an overwhelming urge to put my head down on the table. Next thing I knew I was out cold! Besides scaring everyone in the restaurant and almost ending up in an ambulance (luckily I revived just in time to cancel the one they'd called for me), I learned a very valuable lesson in basic self-care while pregnant: Avoid low blood sugar at all costs!

SLEEPING

Some pregnancy books say that you'll only need eight hours of sleep a night. Don't believe them! Every woman I know needed to sleep an incredible amount during the first trimester. Why are you so tired? First, your body is producing a new human being from scratch, which is very hard work, as well as building the placenta that will nourish it for the next nine months. Second, you're coping with tons of hormones flooding your system, making you a prime candidate for the debilitating effects of nausea and emotional duress. A good analogy is to imagine that your body is working about as hard as it would if you were going mountain climbing—each and every day! You may need to sleep up to 12 hours a night, and take naps during the day as well. And remember that this will not be uninterrupted sleep—your night is likely to be filled with trips to the bathroom and cramming down a snack or two. Only you can decide how much sleep you need, so don't let anyone tell you you're sleeping too much. Spending enough time alone just being calm and quiet is also really important, especially early in your pregnancy. As your pregnancy progresses, you may find that you need slightly fewer hours of sleep over-all, but your days of sleeping through the night are likely over. A good preparation for the early days of parenting to come!

PEEING

Especially during your first and third trimesters, when the growing uterus presses on the bladder, you will feel a very strong and quite frequent need to pee. Don't hold it in, or you may get an infection. Keep your fluid intake up, even if you may be tempted to drink less water to reduce the number of bathroom trips you need to make. You have to pee anyway, so you may as well stay healthy.

WHAT—ZITS AGAIN?

Just when you thought you were a real grown-up and finally rid of zits for good, you may see them return. Outbreaks can occur on the face, back, chest, even shoulders. Blame it on hormones, stay as clean as you can, and try to forget about it. Certainly, if you have a serious skin problem you should see a doctor, but taking any medications for acne during your pregnancy is usually not a good idea. If you are taking medications for acne or other skin ailments when you become pregnant, make sure you tell your provider. You may also find you break out only in the beginning of your pregnancy, and have soft, smooth skin for the rest of it. Other women who never break out may do so now.

Taking Care of Yourself During the First Trimester

Eating for Two

FOOD REQUIREMENTS

One of the hardest tasks of a new pregnancy is learning how to eat properly. Some women are so busy throwing up that the thought of trying to eat better or new foods can be daunting. Indeed, sometimes just getting something down is the most you can accomplish. Yet, dietary improvement in the first few weeks is extremely important. Not only is your own body's need for certain nutrients accelerating, but this is also the time your fetus is developing its entire neurological system. Since lesbian pregnancies are necessarily planned, we have an edge over some straight women, who may continue with bad habits for months before they really accept that they're pregnant. Since we're living in two-week cycles, we can start preparing our bodies for pregnancy each time we begin trying to conceive. This means starting to take prenatal vitamins either while we're trying to get pregnant or immediately after pregnancy is confirmed. I'd recommend taking them while you're trying, but they can be constipating, so you may want to wait. Or you can take a prenatal equivalent with less iron to avoid constipation—but check the amounts of certain components while you are pregnant, just to be safe. For example, you don't want too much Vitamin A in your system, as this can cause fetal problems.

NUTRITIONAL FYI

It can be daunting to look at the nutritional "requirements" that most books and doctors recommend for pregnant women. The amount of food you're expected to eat can seem like more than you could ever consume. You may ask yourself how you could ever eat five portions of protein and five portions of grains a day. Well, the answer is that you won't always be able to, but it's good to see what is recommended and adapt that for your own body. It's best not to panic about meeting every requirement on the food charts you'll be presented with. Generally, if you eat a well-balanced diet, including lots of fruit and vegetables, and then add on extra protein and dairy, you'll be okay. The best thing to do is listen to what your body tells you it needs—and what it wants you to stay away from. However, it's a good idea to review the following information so you can make informed choices.

Keep in mind that if you are carrying multiples, you will have greatly increased nutritional needs, especially for protein.

Things You Need to Eat

- Folic Acid. A very important vitamin for prenatal development. Most prenatal vitamins should include 0.8 mg (800 micrograms), 200 percent of the recommended adult daily allowance. Folic acid is also found naturally in foods such as cantaloupe, oranges, and dark-green veggies like kale, and it is now added to some commercially prepared breads and pastas. It helps prevent deformities such as cleft palate and neural tube defects such as spina bifida, in which the spinal cord grows outside the spinal column.

- Protein. For a pregnant woman, getting enough protein is probably more important than eating enough green veggies. This means about three servings a day of meat, fish, eggs, or cheese. You can also eat tofu and other soy products for protein. If you're a vegetarian, make sure you drink milk and eat yogurt, beans, seeds, and nuts. Talk to your healthcare provider if you're a vegan, as you may need special supplements. Eating protein builds your baby's tissues, and it will also cut down on your morning sickness.

- Calcium. You need about 1,200 milligrams a day—calcium builds the baby's teeth and bones. If you drink milk or eat other dairy foods, you probably get enough calcium. I craved cottage cheese, which made getting enough calcium easy for me. Calcium is also found in dark-green leafy veggies, dried beans, and canned fishes like salmon and sardines.

- Carbohydrates. Forget all the diets currently in vogue that discourage carbs. You need lots of carbs when you're pregnant, and the emphasis should be on whole grains like brown rice, whole-grain breads, and beans and lentils.

- Vitamins and Iron. Eating a well-balanced diet with enough fruits and vegetables (especially dark-green leafy ones), along with a good prenatal vitamin pill, generally ensures that you get enough vitamins. Many women don't get enough iron in their regular diet, but prenatal vitamins should help bridge that gap. If you're a vegan, you should make sure you get enough B12 from the supplement you're taking. Iron helps your blood carry oxygen to the baby. It's also been found that eating or drinking vitamin C–rich foods like orange juice will promote iron absorption.

Foods and Beverages to Avoid

DON'T DRINK THESE

You know that your body needs lots of vitamin-packed juices, smoothies, and especially water when you're pregnant. What shouldn't you drink? First, don't drink alcohol, especially during your early pregnancy. Recent studies have shown that having even a few drinks up until the very last weeks of pregnancy kills brain cells in your unborn child. The dangers of fetal alcohol syndrome are real, and this condition is devastating. Mental retardation, impaired vision, all kinds of behavioral problems, and even stillbirth can result. Alcohol is poison, no matter how the alcohol industry packages it or how good it can make you feel. Would you drink any other kind of poison while you were pregnant? Of course not. If you have a problem with drinking to excess and fear you won't be able to give it up for your pregnancy, get help immediately.

So what about coffee, another drug of choice? Sorry, gals, coffee is pretty bad for your pregnant self and your fetus. The occasional cup o' joe probably won't do any damage, and many pregnancy books say having one or two caffeinated beverages a day won't cause harm. But excessive caffeine consumption, in the range of several cups or more a day, can cause birth defects. Decaf may be a better choice if you absolutely need coffee. Even better, switch to steamed milk in the morning. You'll be getting the calcium your pregnant body needs and you'll feel you're getting your morning fix of frothy hot beverage. Steamed milk is what I drank almost every morning of my pregnancy, and I still find it a relaxing beverage from time to time—as does my now six-year-old daughter. If you're a tea drinker, remember that black teas are caffeinated; herbal teas are a better choice. A word of caution, however: Some herbal teas have abortifacient properties and may cause spontaneous abortion in pregnant women. These include pennyroyal and blue cohosh. Check with an herbalist for more details.

DON'T EAT THESE

Foods to avoid are any that may contain parasites or pose a risk of otherwise poisoning the fetus. These include raw meat of any kind, raw fish and most sushi (order vegetarian sushi instead), raw eggs in salad dressing, some deli meats, and soft cheeses. In your first trimester especially, avoid bitter foods such as broccoli and brussels sprouts. Some doctors believe it is a good idea to avoid the skins of potatoes, which are thought to be slightly toxic. Many herbalists recommend staying away from licorice, sage, nasturtium, celery seed, and ginseng.

Avoid anything you have the slightest aversion to. It's your body's way of protecting the fetus!

And remember, if any food makes you recoil while pregnant, don't eat it! A bad reaction of any kind to food you're considering eating is your body's way of protecting your unborn child. While there may be nothing harmful in that plate you've been presented with, it's your prerogative as a pregnant woman to say no.

KICK THE JUNK FOOD HABIT

There's never a better time than pregnancy to purge yourself of a junk food habit. Do it for your baby, and then rejoice that you also did it for yourself. It is a blessing to take the best care of yourself you can right now, and eating well is top priority. Remember, most of your baby's important neurological development occurs in the first few weeks after conception. If you aren't providing good nutrients to your fetus during this time, you risk causing the baby damage. Deprived of the nutrients needed to develop, the baby will drain off your resources in desperation to get them. This will cause you to feel even more sick than you might already, so do both of you a favor and eat well. Remember, there's a reason why snack items like chips, candy, and soda are called junk food.

Pharmacy Time-out

I hope you'll already be taking prenatal vitamins when you find out you're pregnant. If not, you need to start taking them right away.

But what about the other meds you already take regularly? What's safe to keep taking? What should you discontinue for the duration of your pregnancy? Or while breastfeeding?

This can be a tricky question, since many people think a pregnant woman shouldn't even pop a pill for a headache. We know now that any drug the mother takes, whether recreational or medical, is absorbed through the placenta and right into the baby's bloodstream. This can cause a whole slew of problems, including miscarriage. In fact, many drugs can even prevent a fertilized egg from implanting in the first place.

For women not taking any regular meds, choosing a drug-free pregnancy will be easy. But what if you have been taking prescription medicine? Optimally, you have already discussed this with your doctor or midwife while you were attempting to get pregnant. If not, this aspect of your pregnancy will need immediate and careful consideration, and monitoring by a healthcare practitioner. For example, what if you have been taking a low dose of antibiotics for rosacea? Most antibiotics, such as tetracycline, are not recommended during pregnancy. Do you take painkillers for an injury? Most are considered unsafe in pregnancy. What if you are taking antidepressants, and fear the effects of stopping them? You may hear from your doctor that certain antidepressants are considered safe during pregnancy. You should check the most current research available on this topic. For a first-person account, read Lauren Slater's memoir *Love Works Like This: Opening One's Life to a Child*. After much deliberation and soul-searching, Slater gave up taking her meds for the first trimester of her pregnancy. She captures that experience with great honesty and thoughtfulness in her book, which is also an enjoyable read about a woman coming to terms with the meaning of motherhood.

That Nasty Habit

Do you smoke, or does your partner? When a pregnancy is confirmed, it's past the time to stop. Smoking causes damage to a fetus in many ways, including a propensity for low birth weight, and it may cause premature labor or even miscarriage. Your baby would never choose to smoke—so stop for him or her. Secondhand smoke is also a terrible affliction to an unborn child, so don't let anyone smoke around you or in your house. Do not downplay the serious effects of this hard-to-break habit on your unborn baby. Do everything you can to quit, and use your power as a pregnant woman to urge everyone around you to stop too. Don't worry about offending anyone, whether it's your partner, your best friend, or even your mother-in-law.

You are your child's source of life—if you don't protect your baby's health, who will?

The Full Rubdown

Many women extol the virtues of massage while pregnant. However, you should receive massages now only from someone who is experienced in doing bodywork on pregnant women. Some massage therapists specialize in prenatal massage and really understand a pregnant woman's body. Why is this important? Because certain pressure points on your body should not be worked on while you are pregnant, as this can cause early labor or miscarriage. You should also inform anyone who does acupuncture or any other bodywork on you that you're pregnant.

Hot Tubs and Sauna

In other parts of the world, limited hot-tubbing and sauna use are relatively common among pregnant women. In North America, however, common wisdom holds that both are considered unwise. Your body temperature may rise too high, which could cause you to pass out. One of the hardest things for me in getting pregnant was giving up my weekly visit to Osento, San Francisco's women's sauna. But at the gym after my regular prenatal swims I'd still dangle my feet in the hot tub...ahhhhh. Your healthcare practitioner may feel that a hot tub or a sauna is okay. If so, use tubs in moderation, and don't stay in too long. And make sure to drink plenty of water.

Exercise

Even for fairly active gals, exercise may be the farthest thing from your mind in your first trimester. You will probably feel nauseated and tired. Walking even two blocks can feel like a mile. But the more you can move your body, especially while getting fresh air, the better. The best forms of exercise for pregnancy are yoga, swimming, and walking. Women who have not been especially active before conceiving should at least try to walk every day. Use pregnancy as a good reason to improve your health! Most women can carry on their normal physical activities during the first trimester, as long as you have the energy for it. I know an experienced runner who ran throughout her pregnancy and claimed she was not in discomfort till her last few weeks. Because the baby is cushioned in its sac, it's protected from the jostles of such activity. But make sure to get your doctor or midwife's green light for this first. If you weren't fairly active before you got pregnant, don't get overly ambitious now and embark on a strenuous exercise program. Use good sense, and remember that moderate exercise is the best bet for most women during pregnancy.

Girlfriends—the Emotional Nitty-Gritty

I am the bio mom in our particular family. I was pregnant after the third try, but it took a long time to even believe I was pregnant. Because I didn't have any morning sickness nor many changes in my body other than exhaustion, it was hard for my partner to tell anything was different. Then when I felt the baby kick and she couldn't, she began to feel left out and to get tired of the mind consumption of the pregnancy. My point is, there is that short period when the nonpregnant partner will feel left out, but reality will soon sink in. For us, this happened at around three months when we went to buy the baby's crib. —Fiona

Pregnancy can make the partner of a lesbian become almost completely invisible. I had so many doctors and nurses assuming I was my girlfriend's mother—even though I'm only six years older than she is! It used to drive me crazy! —Ingrid

Pregnancy can cause tremendous stress on a relationship. If you are in a newer relationship, be prepared for some major boat-rocking. If you have made the decision to get pregnant together as a couple, be aware of the stress it can cause for even the best partnership. Most couples weather the storm of pregnancy very well, and many girlfriends become rapt with delight at the baby growing within you. They attend every doctor's appointment, meticulously make you healthy meals, rub your back when you're tired, carry the sonogram picture in their wallet, and cut the baby's cord at birth. Congratulations—you have the perfect second mommy, dyke daddy, or tranny pop by your side! This may be the most exciting shared time of your entire relationship, and you will both be glowing with love.

On the other hand, your girlfriend may not be an active participant in your pregnancy. This is a hard one. It can be traumatic to feel pulled in two directions during your pregnancy. There you are, absolutely excited about and dedicated to the tiny being within. You want to talk about every little change you're going through, and you want to share your excitement and worries with the person you love best. If she's uninterested, it will be upsetting and isolating, and you will wonder how she can actually love you and not also love your growing baby. You may find yourself censoring your excitement so you don't alienate your partner with too much talk about the baby. You may feel that this is necessary in order to keep some equilibrium in the relationship, but it can make you feel resentful and lonely.

To be fair, even the most dedicated girlfriend can feel a bit lost when you are so wrapped up in something she can't feel or see yet. The changes she may witness in you—throwing up and sleeping all the time for example—may be alarming to her. Where did her old girlfriend go? Especially if the pregnancy is more your idea, or you don't live together, or the two of you will not be actively coparenting, she may wonder what her role will be, or even if she'll have one. She may also fear losing you completely after the baby's born.

Because every situation is different, every couple develops their own plan for coping. My advice is to keep communication between the two of you as open and honest as possible. Life is not static, and situations and people change day by day. You may find that your partner becomes more interested once the baby is born and she can develop her own relationship with the new little person in your lives. Or you may find, sadly, that the birth of your child is really the last step in a breakup that's been building for some time. Try to make sure you have emotional support from other people throughout your pregnancy—no matter what happens to your relationship—so you're not left feeling alone during this demanding time in your life.

Legally Speaking

> *My "family" gave birth to our daughter Chloe last year. I am the biological mom, but my partner Anna and I are sharing coparenting (or is it triparenting?) with Chloe's biological father. We all live together in a house we bought. We are in the process of dealing with legal contracts to make sure that Anna is legally recognized as Chloe's parent in addition to me and her father.*
> —Bonnie

> *In the state where we live, there is no second-parent adoption available to lesbian moms. We've had to make sure that we created our own legal documents and agreed to stick to them, even in the event that one day we broke up.* —Melissa

Optimally, you began to lay the legal groundwork for protecting your family before you started inseminating. If not, you will have to play catch-up now. This is especially true if you are planning to coparent with your partner.

NCLR Director Kate Kendell encourages lesbians to do everything they can to protect their families legally. This includes thoroughly discussing with your partner or coparent(s) your shared visions for parenting, and ensuring that you have created the proper agreements. Although Kendell says such agreements may not be upheld in court as "legally enforceable," nor can an agreement force "an unwilling party to be bound by its provisions," in her experience "just having such agreements provides an honor system of checks and balances to families in crisis." This is especially true when the family members who created such documents have "forgotten their original expectations and intent." Such agreements can help in situations where the nonbiological mom is fighting for visitation, and they can allow for the possibility of alimony from lesbian exes. In fact, Kendell says, the NCLR is currently seeing fewer lawsuits involving known donors and more lawsuits

> *It's imperative for the long-term respect of our families that we honor our agreements with each other. If we don't respect our families, the legal system certainly isn't going to.*
> —Kate Kendell

involving lesbian custody—particularly where child support is an issue. The process of crafting such documents, Kendell notes, "demands purposeful attention to the what-if scenarios" that can occur at a later date.

Kendell strongly urges women to pursue second-parent adoptions where available. "They can be vigorously protected" in court in many states, she says. At present, about 25 states (and some Canadian provinces) allow second-parent adoptions, and the list keeps growing. If you live in one of these states and plan to do a second-parent adoption, you should get the ball rolling now so you can finalize your agreement as soon as possible after the birth of your child. Formalizing an adoption may require at least one home visit, several interviews, criminal background checks, an examination of veterinarian records if you have animals, and an appearance in court, and it will cost about $2,000. If you use a known donor, he will have to sever his paternity rights before your adoption can be finalized, so make sure he understands and commits to this from the beginning. The entire process can take up to two years. Consulting a lawyer is the only way to proceed with it.

Couples use other methods to safeguard their families, including wills, a durable power of attorney, and the "Uniform Parentage Act" (UPA), which is currently available in only a few states. Kendell reminds readers that UPAs are relatively untested in the case of lesbian breakups and that second-parent adoption is considered more legally sound. Depending on where you live, you may even be able to get both lesbian mothers' names on a baby's birth certificate. This is tremendously exciting news for women creating families together.

As the issue of queer marriage surges to the front of the fight for equality, it may prove to be the best protector of our family's rights available. Kendell concurs. "While marriage will not solve all issues, it is a readily understood family structure, complete with privileges and protections." Till lesbian marriage is legal everywhere, do everything else you can to protect your family. If you are a single mother, you should designate a legal guardian for your child as soon as you can. If a guardian is not designated and something happens to you, biological relatives will likely be granted custody of your child by the court system.

Not Ready to Coparent with Your Partner?

This is tricky territory, and a subject not often discussed in lesbian circles. Simply put, some women who might be dating or partnered with other women are not coparent material. Or, the relationship might be too new to determine this yet, or even to know whether a coparenting relationship would be desired by either woman. It should also be stated that not every woman who wants to give birth wishes for another person to share equitably the rights and responsibilities of parenting a child. It's best to get these relationship issues sorted out before you proceed with inseminating. If you haven't, and you are now trying to conceive or are pregnant already, and don't feel ready for a coparenting arrangement with your partner, be careful. You may have some sticky times ahead.

Don't promise anything to your girlfriend if you aren't 100 percent sure you want to parent with her. Coparenting is difficult terrain to travel. But if having a baby is your dream, and it is not a dream you have shared and planned as a couple, it's better to parent alone for now. If you're stumbling into legal areas you're unsure of, or you're being pressured by your partner for more than you want to give, talk to an attorney to better understand your options. My own feeling is that it's better to be a happy single parent than to find yourself stuck in a bad relationship with someone who has a growing attachment to your child—and the child to her.

Your Healthy Pregnancy: You and Your Healthcare Provider

Many women find it easy to be out to their healthcare provider. If you didn't come out to your doctor before your pregnancy was confirmed, he or she may assume you are straight. Do both of you the favor of honesty; it will most likely make your pregnancy and your care easier. If you cannot be out to your doctor because of your job, or where you live, or any other reason, at least make sure you are comfortable with the level of care you receive.

If your doctor is blatantly homophobic or makes you feel uncomfortable in any way at all, consider changing doctors early in your pregnancy to ensure continuity of care with the new provider. If you do not have a regular doctor, talk to friends or other mothers in your area, or check an online database of lesbian-friendly doctors for a referral. The Gay and Lesbian Medical Association, at www.glma.org, has recommendations for lesbian-friendly ob/gyns and midwives all over the country. Don't let a fear of homophobia keep you from seeing a healthcare practitioner during your pregnancy. Midwives tend to be easier to deal with than doctors, so if you feel especially anxious about seeing a doctor, perhaps a midwife is the right practitioner for you.

Indeed, you may want to consider hiring a midwife regardless of what your doctor–client relationship is like. In many countries throughout the world, women routinely see midwives for care through their entire pregnancies. In North America, the relationship between midwives and doctors is still a bit shaky. But as midwives gain certification in many states and provinces, more women are realizing that seeing a midwife is a legitimate, woman-oriented approach to prenatal care and childbirth. In fact, midwives were helping women birth their babies long before doctors institutionalized prenatal care and labor. Midwives focus on the physical and emotional health of mother and baby and don't believe in unnecessary medical intervention during pregnancy or birth. The word midwife itself means "with woman," which pretty much says it all. Usually women who are planning home births hire midwives, but even if you're planning a hospital birth, a midwife can be a powerful ally to have by your side.

Unlike the five-minute checkups I had at my HMO, the appointments with my midwives gave me a real sense of the baby growing within me and how to care for it—and myself. When I had a complete emotional meltdown at one point in my pregnancy, midwife Deborah was there to hold my hand and tell me everything was going to be okay. During labor, both of my midwives made sure I was as comfortable and cared for as possible while the baby made its journey through me out and into the world. After the baby was born, they made daily, then weekly, visits to see me and Frances and make sure we were doing okay.

There are midwives in every part of the country, but the standard of care and costs will be slightly different in each region. The services of midwives are generally not covered by any insurance company, but the $1,500–$2,500 typically charged by a midwife is worth it. If you cannot afford this, consider the services of a doula, a professionally trained woman (but without the full range of medical training a midwife has) who supports you during a hospital labor and often cares for you afterward. Unlike most medical doctors, midwives and doulas spend time with you to discuss their services before you hire them. This will ensure that together you make the best team possible for the eventual birth of your baby and your own care afterward. The best way to find a midwife is through word of mouth from other women. You can also look for recommendations online at sites such as www.mana.org and www.narm.org. (See the resources chapter for more information.)

8

You're Well Into It Now!— Your Second Trimester

Welcome to the Golden Trimester

Welcome to your second trimester, which people are fond of calling the Golden Trimester. Whether it's really golden or not I'll leave up to you, but the middle months of pregnancy do seem to provide enough of a break from the weirder moments to allow you to catch your breath.

By now, you're used to thinking of yourself as pregnant, you're not as scared of miscarriage, and you're likely to start showing. People have probably been telling you that you'll feel better now than you've ever felt in your life, but this may be just because you feel more like yourself again after the difficulties of your first few months.

While many of the discomforts of your first trimester begin to fade away now, don't expect a sudden cessation of its worst symptoms. You will probably notice a gradual lessening of morning sickness during the fifteenth to seventeenth weeks, though some women keep waiting... and waiting...for this to happen. Women who say they woke up one day and suddenly felt great may be exaggerating a bit with hindsight. You'll certainly be feeling better, but guess what—there is a whole batch of new things to fret about! Don't worry; the second trimester is also the time to enjoy a renewed sense of energy and joy in your developing baby's

What's Happening in There?

Weeks 13–15 Your fetus has grown to a few inches long and is beginning to look like a tiny human being. It weighs only about three ounces, but it is already growing eyelids and fingernails. It is beginning to develop some muscle tone. Its sex organs are starting to form.

Weeks 17–19 Your baby is about five inches long, has well developed fingernails and toenails, is starting to grow hair, and weighs between four and seven ounces. He or she can blink and move its mouth, and is fairly active. You've put on enough weight that your belly is swelling out, and you will need maternity clothes to stay comfortable now. If you haven't already, you will soon feel the baby move.

Weeks 20–23 Believe it or not, your pregnancy is halfway over, just as you're starting to get used to it. Your baby is already six to ten inches long from head to toe and may weigh up to a pound by week 23. The top of your uterus now reaches your belly button. Your baby's ultrasound photo reveals him or her to look like a small alien, and you may be able to tell its sex. Strangers may notice that you're pregnant now, so get used to the constant questions and comments coming your way.

Weeks 24–28 Congratulations! By week 28, your baby is now considered viable, which means it could be born today and still have a better than 70 percent chance of surviving. The fetus may weigh up to three pounds by week 28 and be over a foot long, and it is covered with vernix, a protective white, waxy substance. Its skin has turned from transparent to more opaque. Your innie belly button may turn into an outie as your belly continues to grow. You will notice the little creature kicking more and more, perhaps especially after you eat or when you lie down at night. The baby can now hear your voice and your heartbeat. You'll find you need to pee often and may have trouble sleeping. For some women, though, this is a period of relative ease, a time when you may regain energy and have a renewed sex drive.

progress. Start deep-cleaning the house and getting everything ready for the baby's arrival. Your due date will be here sooner than you think.

I found my second trimester to be a time for getting things done. Morning sickness was over, I wasn't so tired anymore, and I felt inspired to get everything in order for the baby's arrival. People laughed when I went shopping for the baby this early—they'd say, "You've got lots of time," but I didn't listen, and I'm glad. The weeks will speed by, and the last thing you want to deal with in your third trimester is running around looking for that perfect mobile or changing table. It's also more fun to start buying things and arranging everything now than to wait till the very end.

The Big Payoff—the Quickening

Before you read the litany of second-trimester concerns in the following pages, know that a great moment in your pregnancy awaits you any day now. You will feel a definite movement from within, and you will be reassured to know that there really is a tiny baby in there! This first sensation of the baby's movements, called quickening, can happen anytime from the fifteenth to the twenty-second week. You will probably feel a slight fluttering in your uterus, like the brush of a butterfly's wings. At first, you might doubt that you really felt anything, or you might dismiss it as gas. But soon you will know without a doubt that what you felt was really your baby. Congratulations! You have just experienced one of pregnancy's great milestones, and there's no turning back from here. Soon those flutters will be jabs and pokes at all hours of the day and night. For the next few weeks, these movements will be too small for your partner or anyone else to feel, so right now it's a private party for you and the little one. By the end of your second trimester, others will be able to feel the squirms and wiggles, so get ready for a barrage of requests to feel your tummy.

Medical Tests You Can Expect Now

If yours is a low-risk pregnancy, you won't be given too many tests in your second trimester. You will probably visit your doctor or midwife monthly, and be weighed, have your blood pressure checked, and your urine analyzed. You could be tested for Rh antibodies, which is particularly important in a second pregnancy. You may choose to have several or none of the tests for birth defects and genetic disease (more on this below). Your practitioner will also begin tracking your baby's size, position, and heart rate. If you're told that your baby is lying in the breech position, this means she is feet-first or bum-first. Don't worry too much— babies flip around quite a bit during the second trimester, and this is probably not how he or she will end up. You may elect to take your first ultrasound. If you have the ultrasound after your twenty-third week, you will be able to find out the baby's sex, should you choose to know. If yours is a higher-risk pregnancy, you may get additional tests and monitoring, depending on where you receive care.

Genetic Testing

What Is Genetic Testing?

Genetic tests are given to the mother to determine if the developing baby is at risk for birth defects or any kind of genetic disease. This includes disorders such as Down syndrome, muscular dystrophy, hemophilia, spina bifida, epilepsy, and cystic fibrosis. If you use a sperm bank, you may have been tested prior to insemination for familial diseases such as sickle-cell anemia and Tay-Sachs disease.

Should You Get Genetic Tests?

Some women shy away from genetic testing because they've decided they're "going to have this baby no matter what." That's an honorable credo. However, it's my philosophy that even a bit more knowledge is power. So I tried to balance my anti-interventionist philosophy with the burning need to know if my baby was developing okay. I chose to get all the blood work, and one ultrasound. I didn't feel I needed anything else, given that I was under 35, in good health, and had tested negative for a whole slew of tests at the sperm bank. Of course, this is a highly personal decision, and you may decide you want to take every test available to you. Or you can decide that you don't wish to take any. No doctor or any other practitioner can make a pregnant woman take any tests she doesn't want. Some doctors will advise more testing if you're over 35—the rather arbitrary age that separates what they consider low risk from higher risk. The following sections describe a few tests that are now considered routine prenatal genetic tests.

Chronic Villus Sampling—CVS

The test for CVS is generally optional; it is only given if the mother is older, or has had a miscarriage, or there is a known risk of genetic defects in the family. It is performed sometime between weeks 9 and 13. CVS is, along with amniocentesis, one of the more invasive genetic tests. Actual cells are taken from part of the placenta, either by a tube guided by ultrasound and inserted through the vagina and cervix, or by a needle through the abdomen. There is a risk of miscarriage (1 in 100) and a slight risk of limb or foot deformities in the embryo, since the cells are collected from that region. Results may be ready as soon as a week after testing.

You may also be able to find out the sex of the baby with CVS. The advantage of this test is that it can be done earlier than an amniocentesis or triple screen blood test. However, given the risk of miscarriage, you may choose to wait for the triple screen, described below, unless there are already grave concerns about the health of the fetus.

Triple Screen Blood Test

You'll probably receive a trio of blood tests sometime between weeks 15 and 20. This series is referred to by a variety of names including triple screen, triple panel, and triple marker. The series measures the levels of three substances found in the mother's blood during the second trimester: alpha-fetoprotein (AFP), human chorionic gonadotropin (hCG), and Estriol, a form of estrogen. The levels of these found in the blood reveal the *possibility* of your fetus having Down syndrome and open neural tube defects such as spina bifida. A high level of AFP may indicate spina bifida—or multiples. A very low AFP level may indicate Down syndrome. It's very important to remember that only a fraction of worrisome results from these tests are truly representative of birth defects. These false results can produce tremendous anxiety in a pregnant woman and her partner. Further testing, such as an amniocentesis, will be immediately recommended. Note also that these blood tests cannot check for every type of genetic or birth abnormality.

Amniocentesis

Amniocentesis is an invasive test usually given to women who are over 35, receive questionable results on a blood test, have a family history of birth defects, or a history of miscarriage. It is generally administered between weeks 15 and 17. Earlier than 14 weeks of gestation, amnio carries a 2 percent risk of miscarriage; after 14 weeks the risk drops to 0.2–0.5 percent. It is up to you to decide if having this test sooner is worth a 2 percent risk of losing your baby—the hospital will probably not stress this statistic.

A thin, hollow needle is inserted into the amniotic sac through the front of the abdominal wall, and a small amount of amniotic fluid is withdrawn and used for testing. Some women experience cramping when the needle goes in.

An amnio is not foolproof, but it is over 90 percent effective in detecting neural tube defects and even more accurate in detecting Down syndrome and other chromosomal abnormalities. It also detects the baby's sex. If you are under 35, in good health, and have no family history of genetic problems, there is probably no reason for you to have an amnio. If your amnio shows cause for concern, you will probably see a counselor provided by the hospital to discuss your options at this point.

Glucose Screen for Gestational Diabetes

Many midwives consider gestational diabetes "a diagnosis looking for a disease." It's considered a temporary form of diabetes that develops in women who don't ordinarily have diabetes. If you are generally a healthy eater, you probably won't find this an issue. Help your body cope well with pregnancy by cutting out caffeinated, sugary sodas and junk food. Eating smaller, more frequent meals will also keep your blood sugar levels stable.

Even if a high concentration of sugar is found in your urine, chances are you don't have gestational diabetes. It may simply mean that due to the increased blood in your system while pregnant, you have increased blood sugar. Again, this is nothing to panic about, nor should it mean you are sick or need to take insulin. If you are diagnosed with gestational diabetes, ask your doctor for a thorough explanation of what it is and what it means for you. Only about 3 percent of pregnant women are at risk of needing treatment for gestational diabetes. Often, this is so the baby does not grow too large in utero.

Most doctors perform a routine blood test for gestational diabetes between weeks 24 and 28 of your pregnancy. Prior to the test you'll have to drink a bottle of what tasted to me like flat orange soda. Not pleasant, but not the horrible concoction I'd been warned about. An hour later, your blood will be drawn, and you usually learn the results in a few days. Some hospitals draw blood to test for anemia and STIs at the same time.

Belly Check

At your monthly appointments, to monitor the baby's growth, your belly will be measured externally, with a tape measure, from your pubic bone to the top of the uterus. The measurement in centimeters should correspond roughly to the number of weeks you are pregnant. The baby's heartbeat is also checked. I found it very interesting to see exactly how much my belly had grown.

Physical Changes During the Second Trimester

When I ask if I am fat, I really don't want to know. But when I ask if I am showing, remember, "thick" is the best word. —Tracy

Your Belly Really Begins to Grow

The main physical change of your second trimester is a noticeable growth in your stomach. If you packed on the pounds during your first trimester, you may have already begun to grow a belly, but now is when your tummy truly begins to swell. Most women need maternity clothes now—they're "showing." This is also the time when you may experience a very itchy belly. As your skin swells over your stomach, hips, and back, you may feel incredibly itchy in those areas. Scratching is not the best response, as you may damage delicate skin.

If you have a partner, have her warm up some vitamin E cream in her hands and then slowly and sensually rub it all over your growing parts. Pregnant body worship is always okay!

Many pregnancy books warn against buying special creams for the itching, especially any that claim to prevent stretch marks. However, I found it a real treat to buy myself a special jar of vitamin E cream, which I rubbed regularly on my growing middle. It was much more creamy than plain old drugstore lotion, and buying something special was a small but much-needed luxury. Many women enjoy using these creams. You may also want to try the super-rich cocoa butter creams sold at stores like The Body Shop. Get your partner to enjoy the ritual of taking care of your belly this way. The jury is out on whether such creams help control stretch marks, but your skin will be moisturized, you'll feel pampered, and it will give your partner a way to be involved.

Everything Else Is Growing, Too

Your hair and nail growth are also affected by pregnancy. Your hair may turn thick and grow more quickly now. Even your nails may grow faster, thanks to your hormones. As the ligaments of your midsection stretch to accommodate the baby, you may experience pain in that region. Special support bands can alleviate the discomfort.

Gas and Bloating

It's one of those scary but true facts: Pregnant women get bloated and frequently have gas. There's not much you can do about it other than, as the great kid's book *The Gas We Pass* states, "Fart thee well." Pregnancy is indeed a full-body experience!

Sleep

The constant need to urinate that you experienced during the first trimester may pass by the middle of your second. Which is not to say that you won't still wake up a few times every night. But since your belly is swelling, you may now have a problem finding a comfortable position in which to sleep. You certainly will not be able to lie on your stomach anymore, and some of your other favorite positions won't work either. Many women find that it helps to place a pillow between their knees, or on their side or back for support, or to use one of those special full-body pillows to drape themselves over. I became addicted to one of those during my pregnancy and still enjoy the extra body support they provide. A cushy down comforter

Do whatever you have to in order to get a good night's sleep, whether it be sleeping on the couch or cocooning in a big down comforter. If it means sleeping alone much of the time, so be it.

wedged between your legs and under your stomach is also comfortable. As you near the end of your second trimester, you may also want to begin sleeping more frequently on your left side. This will alleviate pressure on your vena cava and aorta, two major blood vessels supplying blood to the baby. Lying on your side is much better for you than shifting around on your back. When you get into your third trimester, lying on your left side also can be a good way to prevent preterm labor.

Leg Cramps

No one is sure exactly why pregnant women get leg cramps—some suspect a metabolic imbalance such as a calcium or magnesium deficiency. But I can tell you one thing: They sure hurt! They usually strike at night when you stretch out in your sleep. Gently extend your leg out fully in front of you, pointing with your heel, not your toe, into a runner's stretch, and massage it. The tight feeling should pass, though you may feel a bad cramp well into the following day.

Juicy Mama Syndrome

You may notice that you have as much vaginal secretion as you did in your prepregnancy days, or perhaps even more. This is normal, and you shouldn't douche or do anything other than stay as clean as you normally would. My midwife, who calls it the Juicy Mama Syndrome, assures us that it is normal and healthy. Of course, if you have any thick discharge or burning or itching, you should contact your doctor or midwife. You could have a condition such as a yeast or bladder infection, which can be treated even during pregnancy, so there's no reason to suffer the discomfort. You should empty your bladder as often as possible to prevent infection.

Constant Runny Nose

I think I kept the tissue companies in business when I was pregnant, and you may also be wondering why suddenly you're such a drippy-nosed gal. This is called rhinitis of pregnancy. It is caused by the same hormones that are preparing the mucus lining of the vagina for the delivery of the baby; as a side effect you get a nose on overload! You may go through a lot of tissues, but you'll probably find that you don't actually get sick with a cold. If you see blood in the tissue after blowing your nose, it is generally nothing to worry about. If the heat is on a lot in your home, run a humidifier to moisturize the air. This can help alleviate the sniffles and make it more comfortable to breathe.

Hot-Blooded Mama

Being pregnant, you have your own built-in space heater. Even the most cold-blooded among us no longer feel as vulnerable to lower temperatures and minor illnesses. This is partly due to the fact that amniotic fluid, in which your baby swims, is a degree or two higher than your nonpregnant body temperature. Perhaps this is a way our bodies have of protecting our unborn children from chills or disease. In my ordinary, nonpregnant state, I am always the one who needs an extra sweater or blanket at night to stay warm. During pregnancy, I never got cold, and I enjoyed this immensely. Do make sure you dress warmly enough outside, and make sure to stay cool and well hydrated in hotter climates.

Linea Negra

Around this time, many women, especially darker-skinned ones, notice a dark line spreading from their belly button to their pubis. This is called the *linea negra* and usually disappears after you give birth. Why does it appear? Who knows—but you can chalk it up to hormones, like everything else.

Bleeding Gums

Many women experience slight gum bleeding or irritation during pregnancy. It even has a name—pregnancy gingivitis. I found it to be at its worst in the early months. Brushing regularly, especially before bedtime and after meals, should keep this under control, though you may need a softer toothbrush to do so comfortably. Some dental procedures cannot be performed during pregnancy, so be sure to get an appointment for any necessary dental work—as well as a cleaning—before you begin inseminating.

Varicose Veins

About 40 percent of pregnant women get varicose veins, most often in the legs. Your body is producing more blood, and your heart is pumping about 20 percent faster to circulate it all. As blood is circulated through the legs and back to the heart, it pools and creates extra pressure on the veins in the leg. Many families have a strong hereditary predisposition to varicose veins, so they may be unavoidable for some women. While you may not be able to prevent them, exercise when you can, and try to keep your legs elevated while resting. Some women find that rubbing calendula cream on their varicose veins reduces them. These bluish veins can disappear after pregnancy, but are likely to return with subsequent children.

Mask of Pregnancy

Because of hormonal changes, your skin becomes more sensitive during your pregnancy. Any exposure to the sun on your face may result in patches of darkened pigment known as the mask of pregnancy, or *chloasma*. This appeared right across the band of my nose and made me quite self-conscious. Supposedly, it can come back after pregnancy, too, so lather on that sunblock. It may help to bathe in cooler water, avoid drying out your skin, and drink more water so you stay hydrated. My pigment patches disappeared soon after my baby's birth.

Braxton-Hicks Contractions and Early Labor

I'm including this discussion of Braxton-Hicks contractions in this chapter, even though most pregnancy books consider it a third-trimester issue. My first Braxton-Hicks contractions hit solidly in my twenty-first week, far earlier than any woman I talked to at the time. It can be reassuring to know about this phenomenon early on, so if you experience this you don't panic. Think of Braxton-Hicks as your uterus's way of practicing for childbirth. The contractions feel like a small series of lightning bolts or squeezing sensations in your uterus that can move on down to your cervix. They can range from hardly noticeable to slightly painful, and they can really scare you if you haven't experienced anything like them. Braxton-Hicks contractions (named for the doctor who first documented them) are perfectly normal as long as they do not continue for more than a few minutes. If they become really painful or last longer than that, some doctors and midwives recommend that you drink water, lie on your left side, and relax. If the contractions continue, you should call your doctor or midwife: You may actually be experiencing early labor! Drinking eight glasses of water a day is a good preventive for preterm labor.

Shortness of Breath

Because the baby is growing and pushing against your lungs, you may experience shortness of breath, particularly when exerting yourself, even if you're just walking uphill. Press your shoulders back to open your chest up as wide as you can, and try to maintain good posture. Rest when you need to. It's irritating to feel as if you can't breathe, but there's nothing much you can do about it. When your baby is born you'll be able to stride up hills at full clip again.

Heartburn

As your uterus grows, it presses on the stomach, causing stomach acid to back up into your esophagus. This, combined with the already sluggish digestion of pregnant women, can cause heartburn, that burning sensation that spreads across your upper chest and even into your throat. You can take antacids for this discomfort, but most midwives don't recommend antacids because they can block the absorption of calcium. Fresh papaya or papaya enzymes are a safer remedy. Eating more frequent, smaller meals that don't overload your tummy will prevent heartburn, as this will stop your stomach from leaking acid fluid.

Hormonally Speaking

While the horrible mood swings of the first trimester will taper off, your second trimester may continue to be emotionally volatile. The best ways of keeping yourself balanced are ensuring you eat well and get enough rest. Take some alone time whenever you need it, cut back on your work and social schedules if you can, and just pamper yourself! It's amazing what taking a nice long bubble bath while reading a junky magazine can do to ease the spirits. Tell your partner and any other children firmly that this is your special pregnant woman alone time, and make sure they respect it. A lock on the bathroom or bedroom door will also work wonders in promoting personal space.

Shopping

Your second trimester is indeed the perfect time to shop. You have energy, you're excited, and the shops seem to be filled with items you simply have to have. And besides what you need for baby, you need some new clothes for your rapidly growing body. Bring out those credit cards—but don't max them out. What do you really need? Read on.

Maternity Shopping for Dykes

By now, your normally baggy clothes are probably just a wee bit too tight for both you and your ever-growing belly. That means it's time to take the plunge into one of pregnancy's oldest traditions: shopping for maternity clothes. Certainly, we each have our own sense of style, but keep in mind that loose-fitting, all-cotton clothes keep you most comfortable during your pregnancy. Some women refuse to buy maternity clothes at all and just wear really big sizes of their usual duds. This is especially the case for those dykes among us who are more on the butch side. But large sizes of regular-cut T-shirts and sweaters may be way too big in the shoulders, sleeves, and hem if your frame is small. Maternity clothes let your belly breathe while keeping the rest of you in proportion, so it's worth investing in one or two true maternity outfits.

The mall nearest you may sport scary frilly stretchy velour wear that you'd never consider in a million years. And why should you? Happily, in the years since I was pregnant, many large clothing companies have launched more affordable, less appalling maternity lines. Target carries stylish and comfortable maternity basics, much of it very inexpensive. The Gap has a great line of maternity jeans, but you may only be able to find them online. Even Wal-Mart has basic maternity pants, leggings, and shirts. And if you are uncomfortable shopping in a store as a pregnant woman for any reason, including being butch or FTM, online shopping is easier than ever.

Maternity clothes have come a long way, so there's no reason you can't be both comfortable and stylish, no matter what your fashion tastes are!

The old standby for many pregnant women has always been a good pair of overalls. Buy them big so they'll fit through your entire pregnancy. Maternity jeans with a stretchy waist may also be an option. If you normally wear dresses, try some basic loose cotton ones, or spring for a maternity dress, which you can wear with specially cut leggings. I found this very comfy. Smaller-framed women may be able to wear many of their looser-cut prepregnancy dresses throughout most of their pregnancy. Sure, your belly may bulge out a bit, but let it show, girls. There's nothing more sporty than a pregnant belly!

Thrift shops may also harbor surprise finds, items perfect as cheap pregnancy clothes, and do be sure to ask friends who have recently given birth if they have any togs you can borrow for a few months. They'll

Some Safety Tips for
Setting Up Baby's Nursery

- Safety standards have changed, so be aware when using older or recycled items
- Use a crib with slats no more than 2 3/8 inches apart and no corner posts. The crib mattress should fit snugly, and you should not use loose bedding or pillows in the crib
- Keep the baby's crib away from heaters and the cords hanging from window curtains and blinds
- Install a smoke alarm in the nursery
- Don't paint the nursery or install new carpeting right before baby arrives—the fumes may still be toxic

---

probably be happy never to see that shirt they wore for three months straight again. If you have a larger budget, and more feminine tastes, check out higher-end maternity shops like Japanese Weekend (who also have really comfy nursing bras) and Liz Lange. Look for online sites like www.Pumpkinmaternity.com. Even stalwart Lands' End carries maternity now. Many sites promise "cute" or "hip" clothing—unheard of when I had my daughter. You can even buy used pregnancy clothes on sites such as eBay. Even if you are confined to bed rest you will be able to do most of your shopping for yourself and your baby online. Take advantage of this and create your own pregnancy style. No need to be as frumpy as I was.

Some of these sites also offer "transitional" clothing for the time after the baby is born when you still have a fuller figure. Others sell nursing bras, nursing tops, and baby clothes. If you're having a hard time finding bras for your new, heavier breasts in a regular store near you, check a maternity store or some of the online shops mentioned above. Your sensitive breasts need and deserve comfort and support. If you wear an underwire bra, remember you'll need a nonunderwire type for your last trimester, as it's more comfy and won't get in the way of your developing milk ducts.

Taking Care of Other Business

Since you will probably be feeling pretty good during your second trimester, this is the time to take care of other preparations for the baby.

Why wait till you're feeling tired and uncomfortable to fix up the nursery, when you can do all that now and be ready? People teased me about buying diapers when I was only 15 weeks pregnant, but I'm a girl who likes to be prepared. During pregnancy, that's a good motto to have. Go shopping now for some basic necessities like a few boxes of newborn diapers (don't buy too many, as the baby will quickly outgrow them) and other layette essentials. It's also a good time to sort through donations of clothing people have given you, clean out dresser drawers and closets, decide where you'll want to give birth and how, hire a midwife or doula if you haven't already, and think about what other items you'll be needing once the baby arrives. While you're at it, you may want to write up a will or power of attorney, ponder day-care options, and look forward to the accomplished feeling you'll get from taking care of these details now as your due date creeps ever closer.

Remember to wash all clothing and bedding items with a baby-safe detergent like Dreft before using them.

Baby's Layette

Don't go on a big spending spree until after your baby shower, and even then buy sparingly, as the gifts may continue to roll in. Not only that, babies grow very fast, and may quickly outgrow that cute outfit you had to have—before you ever use it. However, you will need a few essentials, and you want to have them ready for the baby's arrival. This includes the following items, in quantities depending on your budget:

- Three to four tiny undershirts or "onesies"
- Coveralls and sleepers
- A few pairs of socks or booties
- One or two sweaters or sweatshirts
- Two hats
- A coat or bunting bag for cooler weather
- Receiving blankets
- Bedding for the baby's crib or bassinet, if you're using one
- Burping cloths
- A baby carrier or sling
- And, of course, diapers

Diapers

Whichever type of diaper you plan to use, make sure you have them in newborn size and one size larger. As for the big debate over whether to use cloth or disposable, consider your lifestyle and budget as well as your desire to help save the planet. Yes, disposables create landfill, but one batch of cloth diapers must be washed multiple times, often with bleach or bleach substitutes. Doing all that laundry burns energy, uses lots of water, and also creates waste. Some people feel that the chemicals used in making disposables so absorbent are bad for the baby's genitals. If you change your baby frequently and don't let the diapers get soggy, this will not become an issue. Personally, I find cloth diapers less hygienic, as the baby literally sits in his own poo and his pee. This aggravates diaper rash. Many larger urban areas offer diaper service, which makes it easier for the committed among us to use cloth diapers. I have many friends who used only cloth diapers and swore by them. If you prefer cloth, there's lots of support for your choice online, and there are many woman-owned cloth diaper businesses to buy from.

Not all disposables are created equal, so try several till you find a brand you like. Huggies quickly became the favorite in my house—they have easy-to-use tabs, they stay on, and they don't leak. Other friends have preferred Pampers and other brands. Generally, with diapers, you get what you pay for, so don't buy the cheapie generics or you'll end up with a diaper oozing baby poop all over you.

Taking Care of Yourself During the Second Trimester

Don't Slip Up Now

Arriving at your second trimester usually means that many of your worries about your pregnancy, including the fear of miscarriage, will be alleviated. When your morning sickness disappears and you start sleeping a bit better, it can be tempting to relax the vigilance you were just getting used to.

While it's important to relax and enjoy your pregnancy, it's crucial that you not slip up now. Keep taking your prenatal vitamins. Remember to eat well and get enough protein, vegetables, and fruits to keep your baby growing well and your own health optimal. Eat lots of fiber-rich grains and drink lots of water to avoid constipation and hemorrhoids.

Remember to laugh, get some exercise, and don't slip back into drinking caffeine or alcohol. Of course, recreational drugs of any kind, including marijuana, are a strict no-no. Your body is your baby's temple. Continue to honor yourself and your baby in the most sacred and healthy ways you can.

Piercings

Pregnancy is not the time to indulge in a new tattoo or piercing. In fact, it's advisable to remove many of your piercings now, especially your belly-button piercing. Nipple rings may become uncomfortable as your breasts grow, and if you plan to breastfeed, it will certainly be easier without plugs of metal in the way. Ariel Gore, author of the very cool book *The Hip Mama Survival Guide,* advises taking out your labia or clit rings. Skin may stretch out and piercings shift, and you may not be able to reach down over your increasingly big belly to clean yourself properly. Since this area may also suffer some trauma in labor, you will want to avoid having the piercings get in the way, or cause you discomfort while you heal from birth. You can put in a temporary filling of plastic fishing line or plastic rings while you're pregnant to keep the piercings open, but as Ariel writes, "I'd consider taking them out early and kissing those piercings good-bye...You can always get them redone after you've finished procreating—once you've experienced labor, the pain of repiercing will seem like amateur stuff."

Exercise Now and to the End of Your Pregnancy

While many women find that their energy level remains high through their entire pregnancy, others are unable to do much of anything from the first trimester onward. Still others may feel fine one day and exhausted the next. Go with the flow of your body's rhythms without forcing yourself, and you'll feel better for it. On the other hand, trying to maintain at least a mild level of exercise is good for you and the baby. This will increase your body's flexibility and introduce more oxygen to your bloodstream than you'll receive by simply lying about. While some days simply walking three blocks can feel like a Herculean effort, you may be able to do a moderate workout on others. I slept most of my first trimester, but went kayaking in my third—go figure! At least stretch at home on the days your energy is lowest—you'll stay relaxed and toned for the extra effort.

As you move through your second trimester, the best choices for exercise are walking, swimming, prenatal low-impact aerobics, and yoga. Prenatal yoga is becoming an increasingly popular exercise option for pregnant gals, and classes are given at many gyms, yoga studios, and even hospitals. Partnered prenatal yoga is something you can explore if your honey wishes to participate.

Stay as active as you can within reasonable limits. It's healthy for both you and the baby, and will keep you in good shape for labor!

Unless you're a pro athlete or have these activities approved by your doctor, the no-no's of prenatal exercise include running, scuba diving, horseback riding, skiing, tennis, and heavy weightlifting. Contact-oriented sports, including karate, basketball, and football, are definitely forbidden. And no sit-ups—stop doing any exercise that works your abdominal muscles.

Personally, I found swimming to be the best prenatal exercise. As your weight and bulk increase, moving around on land may become harder, but in the water, your body feels weightless. No matter how tired and crabby I felt before I slipped into the pool, after a half hour of gliding through the cool water I left refreshed and relaxed. The baby generally slept the entire time, too, rocked by the motion of my body doing all those laps. It was a wonderful treat for both of us, and I wish I could have indulged more often than the two times a week I was able to get to the pool.

Making Birth Decisions

How do you make the big decision about where to have your baby? Often, women have a very clear idea of this right from the start of their pregnancy. While there may be some give-and-take based on a partner's preferences, the pregnant woman must have the final decision about where to give birth. After all, whether you have an involved partner or not, it is ultimately a birth journey involving two people—the birth mom and the baby. Pressure from a partner to have a hospital birth because it is "safer" or to use or not use drugs during labor should be respectfully discussed, of course; but it is left to the birth mom to make a final decision.

By the second trimester, most women know what kind of birth they would like to have. True, one never knows what will actually happen in labor, but you should have a rough idea of where and how you'd like to deliver. Talk to your doctor, midwife, partner, and other women your age who have recently delivered. Most important, listen to your heart. Only you can decide which experience will be right for you. Write up all your ideas about the kind of birth you want to experience and compile them in a birth plan. Making your birth plan will help you formalize these thoughts and will provide a blueprint of your wishes for the hospital staff.

Some considerations for your birth plan include whether you want to be given pain relief and what kinds you prefer, whether you would like to be able to move around during labor and be allowed to take a shower, whether you wish to have an episiotomy, and whether you want to be allowed to eat or drink during labor. Your birth plan may also include a list of the people you want to be present, how long you'd like to wait to cut the cord, who will cut the cord (perhaps your lover or a good friend), what you would like done with your placenta and cord blood, and information about "lying in" with your baby. Stress that you do not want your baby taken away from you after birth unless medically necessary. You may also want to make it clear, if you plan to breastfeed, that you do not want the hospital staff giving the baby a bottle, whether of formula, water, or sugar water. This is frequently done and can hamper early breastfeeding efforts. Your birth plan is best shared with your doctor or hospital staff before labor begins. And understand that even though you have deliberated about every last detail of this plan, you may not be able to actualize any of it.

Choosing a Location

HOME BIRTH

Every pregnant woman wants to have a birth that is safe, not too scary, and not too prolonged. Where is this most likely to occur? Despite what you may think or may have heard, home is the safest place for a woman to give birth. Let me repeat that for you skeptics out there: For a normal, low-risk pregnancy, a minimal-intervention birth in a comfortable home environment is a safer birth. At home, there is less chance of unwanted and unneeded medical procedures being forced on the laboring woman, and certainly it is a more peaceful place for the baby to be brought into the world.

You will not likely hear about home birth from most of your family or friends, and certainly not from the medical establishment. If you are thinking about home birth, educate yourself by reading books on the topic, talk to a home-birth midwife, and know that you are not alone or a freak for considering this option. In fact, in playground and playgroup discussions, most women who had their babies in the hospital express the wish that they had given birth at home. I have engaged in hundreds of discussions with women about their labors, and only a small minority ever expressed real surprise that I survived a home birth without pain meds. Most often I get a wistful reaction, with a comment about how they wanted a home birth but their husband or partner felt the hospital was safer.

My home birth was a wonderful experience, and it was totally manageable without pain medicine. It was very reassuring to be at home with the people I loved and trusted attending to me. The midwives were incredible in guiding me through the experience and gently welcoming my baby into the world. If you have no major complications during pregnancy, home is a natural place to give birth. You get to pace around your own home, have a shower or bath, eat what you want, and go for a walk if you're able. Even if you initially reject this idea, it's an option that you can reconsider as you get close to term. Many women who choose a hospital birth for their first child are more open to the idea of home birth for their subsequent deliveries, because they now know what to expect in labor.

To learn more about home birth, read Sheila Kitzinger's classic *Homebirth: The Essential Guide to Giving Birth Outside of the Hospital*. Even if you aren't considering home birth, this book offers a wonderful perspective on creating a gentle, loving birth environment for both mother and baby. It is currently out of print, but used copies are available online.

HOSPITAL BIRTH

Most women give birth in a hospital. There are various reasons for this. Health insurance may cover only hospital births, ruling out home birth for women who don't wish to pay out of pocket for the services of a home-birth midwife. Societal pressures to have a hospital birth may be very strong. There is an assumption that hospitals are safer than giving birth at home. It's true more medical equipment is available, and this can be reassuring to some people. Partners, even more than the birthing woman, may feel reassured by all this equipment, just as fathers typically are. It signifies to them that "experts" are at hand in case anything goes wrong. Since the birth is largely out of their hands, it may feel safer for them to put it in the hands of the techies and medics. If you choose to give birth in the hospital, make sure to outline beforehand what you do and do not want to happen to you during labor. Consider what is the most intervention you will accept, and what drugs you want for pain, if any. (See the discussion of putting together a birth plan, above.)

You may be able to use the services of a midwife or a doula in the hospital, and I advise you to consider this. A midwife's hands-on powers may be limited in the hospital, but your hospital birth experience will be vastly improved by her presence. Alternatively, you could hire a doula. A doula is a professional labor assistant who provides guidance and support before, during, and immediately after childbirth. Her medical training may not be as extensive as a midwife's, but she is skilled at helping the birthing woman. Often having a midwife or doula present is a good idea for lesbian couples—they can help ward off homophobic attitudes from hospital staff, as well as ensure that you and your partner are respected as a couple and a family throughout the birthing experience. While you are in labor it will be very difficult to concentrate on anything other than getting through each contraction, especially if you want natural childbirth. Having a midwife or doula present to advocate for you and help you deal with your labor is very empowering.

To find a doula, contact DONA, Doulas of North America, at (206) 324–5440 or www.dona.com.

BIRTHING CENTER

My birthing center birth was everything I hoped it would be—just like giving birth at home, but with more space (we were living in a tiny apartment at the time) and a hospital just around the corner in case of emergency. I spent most of my labour in the Jacuzzi with the lights down low. My partner and a friend took turns looking after me, and the midwife checked in every now and then. I used some hypnobirth techniques, but being in water was the best thing of all. The baby was born in the big comfy bed, and afterwards my partner and our child and I all curled up and slept.

We caught a taxi home less than twelve hours after the birth, and
fell asleep together all over again. —Rose

Are you leaning toward a home birth? Would you like to be attended by
midwives but still deliver in the hospital? Then a birthing center may be
the right option for you. Some hospitals have separate wings with a less
institutional setting, and some birthing centers are freestanding. These
will vary in tone and can have vastly different philosophies and rules, so
it's worth visiting a few. Many have hot tubs, showers, and actual, comfortable beds. If you really want to spend part of your labor in the water,
make sure you ask what percentage of women birthing in the center
actually get to use the Jacuzzis. If you're really lucky, your insurance may
cover all the expenses associated with a birthing center labor.

The Birth Certificate

If you are using an anonymous sperm donor, there are several ways you
can refer to the father on your child's birth certificate. Some people use
the term *unknown*, others use *withheld*, which is rather offensive for lesbian families. There may be an option for you to simply have a line typed
across the space for the father's name, as I had done on my daughter's
birth certificate. I felt this solution was preferable to the other terms, which
seemed derogatory or suggested that I couldn't remember who the father
was, or just wouldn't say. Check with your local municipality before your
baby is born, and don't be afraid to fight for your preferred terminology.

When using a known donor, it is best to leave the donor's name off
the birth certificate. Typing his name on the "father" line of the birth
certificate adds legitimacy to his relationship to the child and will be used
in court as proof of paternity if he ever sues for custody. In addition, if the
donor or biological father's name is on the birth certificate, you will have
to provide a notarized form from him every time you want to cross an
international border with your child. This could be a big problem if
you're not in frequent touch with him and need to leave the country,
with or without your female partner. If he will be actively coparenting
and you want to acknowledge him, or if he has simply pressured you to
include him, see a lesbian-friendly lawyer before your baby is born. It is
no easy feat to change a birth certificate later on to exclude him.

Most lesbian couples are able to get the nonbio mom's name added
to the birth certificate after a second-parent adoption goes through. In a
groundbreaking case, a lesbian couple who married in Massachusetts in

June 2004 and had a baby shortly afterward were both named on the birth certificate. This is because state law mandates that married couples who have a child through artificial insemination be recognized as parents. Legal issues that apply to the queer community are changing constantly. Unfortunately, however, as technology races on, bypassing the law, the possibilities for conflict increase in such situations, according to NCLR's Kate Kendell. See a knowledgeable lawyer for advice!

Preparing a Sibling

How you tell your other children and how they react to the news of a sibling on the way depends on their age. Toddlers won't really understand much, even if you prime them with details long in advance. By the age of three, a child may understand there's a baby growing in Mommy's belly but probably won't get interested or jealous till the baby's born. Older children will probably pick up on the changes in you and the rest of the household, so early honesty is the best policy here. In some families, an older child may be included in family decisions and may already know that Mom—or her partner—has been trying to get pregnant. It may be helpful to read together age-appropriate books about new siblings and how babies are

While doing the research for the second edition of this book, my six-year-old frequently could be seen sprawled amidst a pile of pregnancy books. Her favorites are always the ones with graphic photos of birthing women. Far from finding them scary, she is calmly fascinated by them. These books have provoked great conversations about birth between the two of us. When she grows up, she recently informed me, she wants to be a midwife. If I were to have another child, I can't imagine doing so without her being able to witness this tremendous event.

born. A couple of general books on this subject that you might want to check out are *The New Baby at Your House*, by Joanna Cole, and *Za-Za's Baby Brother*, by Lucy Cousins. A beautifully illustrated children's picture book on home birth, from the perspective of an older sibling, is *Welcome With Love*, by Jenni Overend, illustrated by Julie Vivas.

If children are going to be at the birth, they need to be prepared for what they are going to see and hear, and how the laboring woman may act. *Welcome with Love* shows how the mother will have pains in her tummy and describes the birthing experience in just enough detail for little minds to absorb. Older children may enjoy looking at birth photos or books and discussing this with you.

It's highly advisable to arrange for a support person to be available just for the child or children present at birth. Many hospitals have policies about children at births, so inquire before arriving. Some people think that witnessing a birth is not appropriate for preschool children, as it may be too upsetting for them. Home midwives dispute this; they believe a child who is properly prepared will remember this as an incredible experience. Children who witness the birth and find it a positive experience are more likely to welcome a new sibling rather than treat it as an intruder who came from the hospital. A friend of mine who had a home birth had a special adult friend paired with her son for the labor. By late evening, her son was tired out by all the excitement and ready to go to bed. The labor went on all through the night, and five minutes before his new sister emerged into the world, he somehow managed to wake himself up and come quietly into the room to watch.

How did he wake up in time to do this? Home-birth magic, many would say.

Partners Become Pregnant, Too

It is during the middle trimester that a pregnancy becomes noticeable and therefore "real" to other people. If you are a pregnant woman with a lover who has been part of this process, her interest will sharply increase right about now. Physical evidence that the baby is present and thriving will bring her even closer into the process. For a couple who have planned a family together, there may be no greater joy than to realize that the baby is growing and changing and will soon join the two of you in the world. A partner may start carrying a sonogram photo in her billfold, or singing to the pregnant woman's belly. She will love to feel the baby's kicks and rolls, and allow herself to become more attached to the new creature in other concrete ways.

When Partners Aren't So Supportive

On the other hand, some partners are not so supportive. As anyone who has been pregnant knows, the experience is so all-consuming it may be hard for anyone else to get as wrapped up in it as you. A partner may be looking forward to the baby's birth but can't understand your hormonal mood swings, tiredness, or sudden psychotic need for chocolate. Your partner may wonder where the fun girl she knew prepregnancy has gone—and wonder whether she'll ever reappear. Luckily, pregnancy lasts only nine months, and the joys of family life and parenthood last forever.

If Your Life Circumstances Change

Unfortunately, the relationship with my girlfriend started to go downhill as soon as I got pregnant. I wanted someone to take care of me and while she was supportive of my desire to get pregnant, she was not there for me when I did. Being in such a relationship provided an emotional roller coaster for my entire nine months, with my partner threatening to leave almost monthly. She eventually did soon after my son was born. I'm not sure how I ever got through all that. —Frankie

There is no great time to lose a job, move cross-country, have a parent die, or break up with a girlfriend. But life has a way of throwing us challenges that we somehow manage to cope with. Coping with big life changes during pregnancy is even harder, however, because you are already dealing with a full plate of emotional and physical changes. The everyday blues can be cured by exercising, keeping friends close by, finding a support group on or offline, taking lots of baths, burning candles, writing in a journal, and learning as much as you can about the growing baby inside you. But for life's big heartaches, such as breaking up with a girlfriend, professional counseling may be the best way to cope. Remember that the optimal state of your pregnancy is anticipation, not stress, anxiety, or mourning.

Keep in mind from the start that very few of us have absolutely blissful pregnancies, since during those months (and the time spent trying to conceive) you do not live in a bubble. Some pregnancies occur just as a loved one dies, and it will not ease the pain when well-wishers point out that your pregnancy is part of the great cycle of life and death. What will help is time, and taking care of yourself in the meantime to the best of your ability. Relationships sometimes fall apart from the combined strain of trying to conceive and getting through the many trials of pregnancy. If this happens to you, know that you're not alone, look for a different kind of support system or create one for yourself, and trust that events happen for a reason and work themselves out in the end. Once your baby is born, your hormones will settle down, you'll be back in your old body (or something similar), and you'll have a baby whom you love and who adores you. Though you hurt now, life is bound to start looking up again soon! And don't worry that the normal mood swings of pregnancy might affect your baby negatively. I cried a lot during my pregnancy and, luckily for me, I had the happiest baby anyone could wish for!

Sliding into Third

You have reached the end of your second trimester now, and all signs look good. You are well past the midpoint of your pregnancy, and in only a few more weeks you will be holding your brand new baby! Read on for information about the home stretch of your pregnancy and how to survive those (uncomfortable) final weeks. But first, some much needed information about self-esteem and sexuality during pregnancy.

Self-Esteem and Sexuality During Pregnancy

Why This Book Is Different

If you've read other pregnancy books, you know that information on self-esteem and sexuality issues is scanty. Most of them include a page at most about sexuality during pregnancy, and it's all geared to heterosexual intercourse. Perhaps there will be a few illustrations of "safe" positions for straight sex. Nothing at all on lesbian sexuality, and not much on body and self-esteem issues, either. Not much on how pregnancy changes our very essence, the way it changes how we live in our skin. Why this big silence on sexuality during pregnancy? Why so little discussion about how we relate to our partners during pregnancy, how they relate to us, and how we can better come together? Why is it so hard to get answers about what sexual activities are safe for lesbians? At this point you may rightly be asking, Will sex hurt the baby? And can it start labor?

Desire During Pregnancy

Trying to conceive is a stressful time. Your body may let you know you're about to ovulate by a marked increase in sexual desire. But for the rest of your cycle you may be so stressed about the conception process that you lose your normal sexual feelings. Once you're pregnant, your desire for sex may vary greatly. Some women lose desire completely, some experience a boost in libido, and others experience their very first orgasms. Still others notice no change in desire. Whichever way your sex drive veers, you'll certainly notice the effects of increased blood flow to your genitals. You may feel swollen or uncomfortable, notice more discharge, or be aroused by all the blood pulsing down there. This can lead to a heightened sense of awareness of what's between your legs!

If you are one of those women who experience normal sexual appetite or even an increase in desire during pregnancy, you're very lucky. You may not understand what the big deal is here, because you assume it's the same for all women. If that's your story, slap on the red lipstick, stick that luscious belly out for all to see, and revel in the power of your pregnant self.

> When the urge hit during pregnancy, I wanted it then and there. I even had the urge the day our son was born. —Justine

> During my first pregnancy, especially toward the end, my sexual desire really increased. It was a really great time. Both my partner and I were hoping it would be that way during the second pregnancy. Unfortunately, it wasn't. I guess it was just a different mixture of hormones. —Kayla

> My own sexual urges were greatest when I was about six months pregnant, but my partner wasn't always willing to oblige. At the end, she wouldn't have sex with me at all. I was frustrated and couldn't see what the big deal was. I think she was scared of hurting the baby. —Nanette

> When I was about five months pregnant, an old boyfriend showed up and stayed for a few months until the baby was born. Sex for me was quite enjoyable with him, right up until the end! —Christine

Not Everyone's So Lucky

From talking to hundreds of women during the course of the research for this book, it became clear to me that the experience of most women, whatever their orientation, was that sexual desire tends to dip during pregnancy. This can be due to fear, nausea, hormones, and the way your body is increasingly morphing into some strange other creature.

Sex during pregnancy...what's that?! —Miriam

My sex drive disappeared entirely while I was pregnant. My first trimester was spent feeling nauseous every night, so who'd want to jerk and jolt around! By the time the nausea finally left, it seems like my hormones were on a roller coaster and I was just too exhausted. In the latter part of my pregnancy, my doctor cautioned me against rigorous sexual activity. I had to laugh, given my nonexistent sex life! —Debbie

Physical Changes Could Affect Your Desire

During the first trimester, most women experience some degree of fatigue and nausea. Morning sickness is not exactly a terrific aphrodisiac. Neither is the overwhelming urge to rest, which might strike during the evening hours, when you used to be frisky. If you're going to bed for the night at 7 P.M., sexual activity is obviously not going to happen in the evening. Further erasing sex from your mind might be tender breasts, itchy skin, and acne breakouts. You might also start worrying about whether and how sex will affect your developing baby, even though this concern is usually unfounded. These hormonal and physical changes and your concerns surrounding them are very normal.

My wife and I have always had a very active sex life. But what with me puking for the first four months and the bad smell coming from my cooch in the last few months, neither of us was really in the mood. Plus, I'd just had a miscarriage and didn't want to do anything that could even possibly hurt this one. —Julie

As you move into the second trimester, your morning sickness likely decreases. Your desire for intimacy will ebb and flow, but as your belly swells, you'll really be aware that there's more of you than there was before. Feeling your body grow, noting the baby kick inside you, dealing with strange cravings, and floating along on a sea of hormonal shifts may make it hard to abandon yourself to the realm of sexual pleasure. As you get bigger, you'll feel more awkward in bed, and finding comfortable positions for sex and sleeping will be difficult. To add to the confusion, your partner may be unsympathetic about these changes, and she may even find your luscious new pregnant body a turn off.

Indeed, Anne Semans, a mom who has written extensively about women's sexuality in many books, including *The Good Vibrations Guide to Sex* and *The Mother's Guide to Sex*, says that the "biggest issue for all pregnant women is total loss of sexual desire." She knows of some women who have increased desire, but they are few and far between. As Semans says, "In pregnancy, you're dealing with your own body's changes. It's hard to keep up your sexual self-esteem."

Sexual Self-Esteem

What, then, is a girl to do?

First, be aware that these changes are normal. After spending so many years in the same body, with fairly predictable moods and rhythms, you can be caught off guard by pregnancy. Hormones can sweep over you in a mighty wave, turning you into a hysterical, weeping creature. Put this in perspective by remembering that you haven't always felt like this, and that pregnancy doesn't last forever.

When things feel out of control, go for a walk, spend some time alone, or engage in a pleasant activity with your partner (perhaps a trip to a bookstore, some light gardening, shopping for baby clothes). Take a bath, chat online with other grumpy moms-to-be, buy yourself some flowers. If you're a single mom, make sure you find another expectant mom to talk to so you know you're not alone. Consider getting a massage from someone experienced in prenatal body work. Learn to feel comfortable in the skin you're temporarily in. Support groups for expectant lesbian moms are great places to discuss your concerns about body image and sexuality.

On a personal note, I wish I had enjoyed my sensuality more as a pregnant woman. If I were to do it again, I would put on sporty outfits, wear bright lipstick, and show off my belly as much as I could. If I were partnered, I'd make sure it was with a person who found pregnant women sexy and felt they deserved a lot of pampering. Instead, I wore schlumpy clothes and felt fairly nauseated and exhausted the entire time. And because I was in a rather unsupportive relationship, I wasn't made to feel as gorgeous and special as a pregnant woman should. The lack of empathy and special care during my pregnancy probably had a lot to do with my almost nonexistent sex drive during that time.

Attention, Partners!

Hey nonbio moms, dyke dads, and tranny pops out there: This is a special message to you! Now is the time to reassure your partner that she is more beautiful and more loved by you than ever before. You can't feel the effects of her body's changes, though you can see them starting to happen. Similarly, you won't know how hormones are making her feel crazy, though you might agree she is losing her mind. Being pregnant is difficult work, and you have a job to do, too. Your pregnant partner may be the star of this drama, but you have the main supporting role. Let her know she's a queen, the most beautiful pregnant creature ever to roam this planet. Bring her flowers. Rub her shoulders for her. Do the laundry. Cook her dinner. Listen to her litany of complaints, though you've heard them all before. Admire her curvy hips, those swelling breasts, that belly glowing with life. Even if you're freaked out and think she looks like a scary swollen beast, don't tell her. If you want sex and she doesn't, try to understand when the answer is no. You can always masturbate—together, if you like.

Anne Semans suggests that girlfriends of moms-to-be "show the initiative without putting pressure on your partner." Have a sensual bath together, then lead her to the bedroom and massage her gently. Communication and compromise are important in any relationship, but adoration is even more important right now. If she feels safe and loved, she's more likely to open up sexually, even if she's tired. Boost her self-esteem by letting her know she's doing an amazing job of building your baby. Tell her she's treasured, and you'll both feel better for it.

Cherish Intimacy

While I didn't want sex, I wanted my lover close by all the time. I wanted to be held, petted and cherished. —Carlotta

Actually, I felt more amorous through most of my pregnancy than I did beforehand. I definitely felt more sensual and emotionally open to my partner. —Sharon

Pregnant women do crave intimacy, even if they aren't up for full-blown sex. An emphasis on the pleasure of touch rather than achieving orgasm may help keep you and your partner close. Well-known sex educator and mom Susie Bright suggests that couples focus less on positions and advocates that pregnant women receive "lots of tenderness and passion" during their pregnancies.

Even if you don't feel like being sexual with your nonpregnant partner, you can stay close. Be appreciative of how well she's taking care of you. Include her in the decision making and encourage her to come to your prenatal appointments. It's very easy to get so wrapped up in your pregnancy that you forget she's going through changes too. Talk about your feelings and offer her as much physical touch and emotional support as you're able.

Bright writes eloquently about sex and intimacy in the essay "Egg Sex" in her book *Susie Bright's Sexual Reality*. She claims no woman ever really loses all interest; we're just consumed by our emotional and bodily changes. Documenting her own clit's growth while she was pregnant, Bright says that she couldn't even masturbate the same way anymore, let alone make love in the same fashion. "Your normal sexual patterns don't work the same way anymore," Bright writes. "Unless you and your lover make the transition to new ways of getting excited and reaching orgasm, you are going to be very depressed about sex and start avoiding it altogether."

Try Something New

Toward the end of my pregnancy, some positions got a bit awkward, but generally improvisation worked well. It helps enormously if you have a partner who is turned on by pregnant women. Mine was, and boy was I lucky! —Tammy

Anne Semans also suggests trying to think of sex in a different way during pregnancy. How to do this? There's room for experimentation, and now is a good time to drag out those books on sensual massage or Tantra. Try reading erotic stories or watching some porno together, if you're open to those activities. Here are some other ideas:

- Read sex guides such as the *Kama Sutra* that focus on different types of sexual and spiritual expression

- Explore the world of lesbian pornography
- Try sensual massage
- Read each other erotic stories from anthologies like the annually published *Best Lesbian Erotica* series
- Masturbate alone or together
- Have a romantic dinner out or a weekend getaway
- Share a candlelit bubble bath
- Plan a surprise that doesn't focus on the baby
- Write each other a love letter
- Enjoy letting your daydreams get raunchy

Chasing the Big O

As I stated earlier, your genitals will change during pregnancy. Increased blood flow to your sexual organs could mean your labia feel swollen, or you notice a pulsing in your vagina. If you are able to have orgasms, they may be longer and more powerful. Women previously unable to climax may be able to do so now. Others may find sex uncomfortable, with excitement building quickly and an orgasm staying frustratingly out of reach.

> In comparison to having sex when I wasn't pregnant, I felt my orgasms were now much more intense, but it took more work to get there. —Arlene

Masturbation is one way to relieve sexual tension, alone or with your partner. If you're up for sex play but don't want to be touched, you can always pleasure your partner. Try to relax and not be shy about the changes in your body. When you feel confident and sexy as a pregnant woman, you're more likely to get off.

Lesbian midwife Deborah Simone says that a good, hearty session of sex may be just what a pregnant gal needs. Since pregnancy can be a time of lowered inhibitions, increased hormonal flow, and powerful fantasies and dreams, it can be a great time to explore sexually. Simone recommends staying away from deep thrusting into the vagina, but she suggests making love doggie style, with the pregnant woman penetrated from behind. "This is also a great way to get your perineum massaged," says Simone.

For the truly sexually adventurous, pregnancy and the preparation for childbirth present opportunities for expanding your sexual consciousness.

Susie Bright even suggests thinking of birth as the ultimate sexual experience. While this may not prove to be your experience (it certainly wasn't mine!), don't lose sight of yourself as a sexual being during pregnancy.

Your Sexual Questions, Answered

Here are some answers to specific questions you might have about sexual activities during low-risk pregnancies. If your pregnancy has been classified as high-risk in any way, err on the side of caution during your sexual play.

Is sex safe during pregnancy?

Yes, sex during a normal, low-risk pregnancy is safe. The activities that most lesbians engage in, including touching one another's genitals, penetrative sex with fingers and dildos, anal sex, and oral sex, are not likely to cause problems. Nor is sexual activity likely to cause you to miscarry or go into labor prematurely.

Is it okay if my lover lies on top of me?

In early pregnancy, this shouldn't be a problem, unless your breasts are too sore. As a pregnant woman's belly swells, it will be uncomfortable for her to bear the weight of her partner. In fact, this position may become comical, with that big belly commanding center stage. Try lying side by side, or put the pregnant woman on top.

Is vaginal penetration okay?

Penetration with fingers is considered quite safe. Penetration with dildos and penises is safe in low-risk pregnancies. Although the baby is protected inside your uterus, avoid vigorous hard thrusting with sex toys. Change angles to avoid bumping your cervix. Stop or take a break if you get uncomfortable. Make sure all hands and toys are clean.

What about anal penetration?

Anal sex is safe as long as you proceed carefully. No hard thrusting is advised, and stop if it hurts. Start small: a finger inserted while your partner lies behind you, a small butt plug, a slender dildo. Tristan Taormino, in her book *The Ultimate Guide to Anal Sex for Women,* writes, "It is safe to have anal sex if you are pregnant, although some women find that they cannot get in a comfortable position for anal stimulation." Taormino suggests that pregnant women be extra careful about preventing bacteria from traveling from the anal area to the vagina. Keep sex toys fastidiously clean, including ones you only use in the vaginal area, and always use lube for anal penetration.

Is it okay to use lube for sex play?

A water-based lube is fine for vaginal or anal penetration. Don't use oil-based lubricants in your vagina.

Will sex hurt the baby?

We didn't have much sex when my girlfriend was pregnant, mostly because of me! A twins pregnancy is considered high-risk, and I was so worried that we might do something that would hurt the kids, despite our great ob/gyn's blessing to go right ahead! —Elise

Sexual desire accelerated for me during pregnancy, but because of a past miscarriage, my partner and I were very nervous about sex. We had lots of sex while I was pregnant, but it was much more gentle sex, with limited vaginal penetration. The pregnancy was so precious to us that we didn't want to do anything that might jeopardize it. We had no formal advice on this and certainly wouldn't have felt comfortable discussing this with our doctor.
—Jana

Many pregnant women instinctually shy away from sexual activities that may harm the fetus. According to Anne Semans, that's probably a good thing. "If you're worried about a particular sexual practice, don't do it," she says. "Now is the time to err on the side of safety. One good fuck isn't worth the price of a baby."

While it's true that the baby is protected inside you within the uterus, there are a few sexual activities to avoid. No very deep thrusting of dildos or any other objects into the vagina. Anything that can damage the cervix is also off-limits. This includes any rough sex and all fisting. While cunnilingus is generally fine, blowing air into the vagina is a big no-no. This can create an air bubble in the bloodstream called an air embolism, which can be life-threatening to the mother. This is a rare condition; your partner will not trigger it by breathing normally when she is down there.

More About Rough Sex

Even the most sexually adventurous dyke among us should curtail S/M activities that involve impact (such as whipping or paddling) during pregnancy. (Activities like role play, very light bondage, and the use of blindfolds are, of course, safe.) Additionally, any sexual play that can constrict blood flow, cause cramping, or cause trauma should be ruled out immediately. If you are into extreme bondage, piercing, cutting, whipping or other such activities, take a break from them during your pregnancy.

What about infection?

Vaginal discharge itself doesn't necessarily indicate a problem, and pregnant women tend to produce more than the usual amount. But if you notice a burning sensation, itchiness, or weird smells from your vagina or around your labia, get it checked out by a doctor. Make sure whoever is treating you for this or any other medical problem is aware that you are pregnant—some medical treatments and remedies are not safe for you or your fetus. When you use the toilet while pregnant, be especially careful to wipe from front to back.

What if I get an STI while pregnant?

While STIs (sexually transmitted infections) are never pleasant, acquiring one while pregnant is even more awful. Not only will you be extra embarrassed, you'll find out that many STIs and their treatments can harm your baby—many medications for STIs are so toxic they are not even usable if you're pregnant. It is therefore best to err on the side of caution if you are sexually active while pregnant. Practice safer sex if either you or your partner is not monogamous, or if you are with a new partner whose sexual history is unknown to you. You will probably be tested at least twice during your pregnancy for STIs. If these tests are not required, you might consider getting at least one round just to make sure. If you are found to have an STI, discuss treatment options with your doctor.

Can sex cause labor?

Orgasm always seemed to bring on contractions for me, and on the advice of my doctor, I had to lie with my feet up against a wall until they subsided. —Lee

For the most part my breasts were too sensitive to touch, but my midwife told us that a little nipple play at the very end of my pregnancy could help me go into labor. —Suzi

Sexual play can kick-start your labor—but only if your body is ready for labor to begin anyway. In a low-risk pregnancy, it's okay to be sexual, as long as you haven't been given instructions not to play. If you're lucky enough to be feeling sexual, it's okay to go with it, as long as you follow some basic guidelines. Feeling some contractions after sex, especially as your due date nears, is normal. Lie down and rest until they stop. You might even feel the baby move as you and your partner have sex. This may make you anxious, but be assured it's normal.

Sometimes, straight women at their due date are encouraged to have penetrative sex with their male partners to bring on labor. This is because semen contains prostaglandins, which can cause the uterus to contract. Penetrative sex with toys won't have the same effect. Breast stimulation can also cause contractions, as well as some leakage from your nipples. In fact, nipple play or other hanky-panky during a stalled labor can get things going again, as it releases the natural hormone oxytocin, which stimulates contractions.

In a high-risk pregnancy, follow your doctor's or midwife's advice about sexual play, and refrain if necessary to prevent premature labor. If you bleed, lose your mucus plug, or your water breaks while you're having sex, stop and notify your care provider.

Ask the Right Questions

If you have concerns or questions regarding sex during pregnancy, it is up to you to initiate a conversation with your healthcare provider. Very few physicians are knowledgeable about the specifics of lesbian sex and sexuality in general, and even less about sex during pregnancy. As an example, if a doctor advises you not to have sex, does this mean only penetrative sex? What about oral sex? What about orgasms? Be prepared to ask explicit questions.

During the first trimester of my pregnancy, I started spotting after an orgasm. I was put on oral progesterone and was told not to have sex. I didn't know if this meant only no penetration like in heterosexual sex, and I wasn't comfortable enough to ask specific questions of my doctor. So I ended up not having much of a sex life during my pregnancy. —Diane

Instead of giving up on sex because you're scared of the unknown, empower yourself with some sex-positive information and support. Talk to other pregnant women about their experiences, have a nice chat with a sympathetic doctor or midwife, and read a book like *The Mother's Guide to Sex* by Anne Semans and Cathy Winks for more information and inspiration.

Chapter

10

Into the Home Stretch— the Last Trimester

Congratulations to You!

Congratulations on making it this far into your pregnancy! The good news is that for the first time, the end is probably in sight, and the months behind you will be starting to blur. Was it really you who was puking into the toilet each morning and craving apricot nectar every afternoon? How pathetic those symptoms may seem now!

I remember my last trimester as a time when everyone kept telling me how excited I must be, and all I wanted to do was to punch them out. Sure I was excited, but I was sick of pregnancy, I could barely move, and I couldn't even see my swollen feet, let alone my vagina. It's natural to become crabby toward the end of your pregnancy, especially if the weather's hot. In fact, you'll know labor is close when you have strange, sometimes violent urges to hurt everyone around you. No joke—the week I went into labor, I even called my midwife to ask if this feeling was normal. She assured me that it was, and that labor was near.

But what really defines your third trimester—weeks 29 to 40—is how big your baby is starting to grow now. If you thought you were large in your early months, you'll be amazed at how much bigger you get during these weeks. Is this really still your body? Yes, but you are a hotel for two (or more) at the moment. Seeing how much your skin can stretch is truly amazing!

Particularly in your last few weeks, your baby will be gaining about eight ounces a week. This, for you, may equal about a pound a week. You may feel there is simply no more room left inside you, and you'll have the symptoms to prove it!

The best thing to do in your third trimester is to relax. If you're still working now, take some time off. Load up the freezer with food. Go for walks to keep yourself limber, but have friends help you out with errands.

> As your partner's pregnancy progresses, you as a coparent will feel more involved. You may even get some of her pregnancy symptoms, such as nausea and backache, like I did. And when she hits month eight of pregnancy, you will be the most important person in her life because without you, she won't be able to scratch her toes or pick up a sock. —Karin

> My belly got really big, and my partner and I would lie in bed with our hands on my belly just feeling the baby in there and watching her move. —Vanita

Most of the ailments and complaints of the third trimester result from this one fact: The baby is growing ever larger. Your uterus now extends from your rib cage down to your pubic bone. It has increased to 500 times its original volume. In it lies a baby, often rolling around, kicking you, and edging into final position. A very common complaint during this time is shortness of breath; it is caused by your uterus pushing your diaphragm into the space usually reserved for your lungs. You may be experiencing vaginal pains as the baby presses down, hip and back pain, heartburn, and occasional urinary incontinence. You may also be suffering from hemorrhoids, those dilated, twisted blood vessels in and around your rectum. If you notice pain, itching, or even some bleeding when you poop, you may have them. The best remedy for hemorrhoids, as well as the best way to prevent them, is to try to keep your stools soft by eating enough fiber and drinking lots of water, and don't strain on the toilet.

You may notice that your energy level swings from high to low one day to the next. Many women experience a rush of energy in the very last weeks, which helps them prepare for the baby's arrival. You may be overcome with the need to hang curtains or put the changing table

What's Happening in There?

Weeks 29–32 Your baby already has all the hair it will be born with. He or she is now about a foot long and can see enough to know whether it is light or dark, and can recognize your voice. If your baby were born a preemie at 30 weeks, odds are good that he or she would survive just fine.

Weeks 33–35 The baby is inhaling amniotic fluid to practice breathing, and you probably feel it when he or she gets the hiccups. Your baby is gaining a lot of weight now and may be settling into a head-down position.

Weeks 36–40 Now you're finally in the home stretch! The baby is continuing to grow, and by the end of week 37 it is considered full term. Your belly will feel huge, your skin will be stretched to the limit, and you may become really cranky. Finally, your baby is almost ready to be born!

---

together. This nesting urge is nature's way of ensuring that you'll have everything in order before the big day comes. Just don't overdo it too close to your due date. You want to make sure you have plenty of energy for your labor!

Taking Care of Yourself During the Third Trimester

The Weight We Gain

Although, as women, we are often force-fed messages encouraging us to stay skinny at all costs, it is healthy to gain weight during pregnancy. It is normal for a woman carrying a baby to gain between 20 and 35 pounds. Some women gain less, and some, especially women carrying multiples, gain more. This will depend on your body type and metabolism, your prepregnancy weight, and of course what you eat. Pregnancy is certainly not the time to diet, because you have an extra nutritional need to nourish yourself and the growing baby inside you. But no matter how much or how little weight you gain, you are sure to hear comments about "how much weight you've gained." This can be very troubling for women who are not sure how to respond or are sensitive to such comments.

First, be aware that not all the weight you gain during pregnancy is due to your snacking. It's important to know why you are gaining a healthy amount of weight, and it will also help you know what to say if anyone is critical of you. You can explain to any detractors that the placenta you have grown weighs about two pounds, your breasts have grown and packed on a couple pounds in preparation for breastfeeding, and your uterus has greatly expanded and grown by another two pounds. If they want to hear more, tell them you're carrying two pounds of amniotic fluid around your baby, who probably weighs between six and nine pounds alone. Not to mention the increased volume of blood in your body, six or so pounds of fat and muscle, and a couple more pounds of fluid. You can let them know it's hard work growing new organs, pumping more blood, and building a new human being from scratch. Finally, tell them that the 20, 30, or 40 pounds you've gained has been an absolute act of love to provide the very best first home possible for your new baby. I guarantee they'll never be rude to another pregnant woman or see her as "fat" again.

Childbirth Classes

We were one of two lesbian couples at our birthing class. Nonevent. The biggest thing I got from the classes was helping to understand the changes the body goes through in labor and the effects of different types of drugs you may be offered so you can make an informed choice. —Betty

My partner and I are taking the classes once a week for six weeks, and we are the only lesbian couple. We also stand out in other ways because my partner uses a wheelchair and we are expecting twins! So we are unique, but the other couples are completely unfazed by us, although I'm sure we're the topic of conversation away from class! But the good thing about being in a class setting is that questions are asked that I wouldn't think of. Also, because I want everyone at the hospital to know just who we are beforehand, so there will be no surprises on delivery day.
—Jennifer

If the idea of attending a traditional hospital class surrounded by straight strangers pushes your comfort limit, here is an idea that worked in our community: ask your caregiver if she is willing to approach her other lesbian clients about a lesbian childbirth series. Voila! Your own cozy class and an instant support system!
—Phoebe

My partner and I took a hospital tour with five other couples, all straight. The tour leader kept saying "you and your husband" despite our obvious lesbian presence. Afterwards, I took her aside and asked if she might use the word partner. She was surprised by my request, as if she had never seen a pregnant lesbian before. Hopefully, she'll remember meeting us next time she sees two women together on one of her tours. —Alice

Taking some sort of childbirth classes is standard fare for most pregnant women. First-time moms especially will draw comfort from a setting where the topic of birth is discussed in detail. These classes generally focus on breathing techniques, different body positions, medications to manage pain, the concept of relaxation during labor, and possible complications that may arise in birth. They are a good opportunity for couples to prepare together for a team approach to labor. For single moms, it's a chance to get in sync with your birth coach. For both single moms and couples, it's a chance to renew your commitment to the person who will be supporting you in labor.

Usually you take childbirth classes a month or so before your due date, so that the information you learn will be fresh in your mind when you start labor. Many women assume they should take childbirth classes in a hospital, but that is not my recommendation to you. Hospital birth classes are often taught by an employee of the hospital, not an independent childbirth educator. If you take a class in a hospital, you'll be learning about birth from someone with a vested interest in that hospital's policies and procedures. If you can, take private classes taught by someone who really cares about laboring women, like classes offered in a neutral environment like a local community center, which encourages freer discussion among the participants. Or, take private sessions from a midwife, if you prefer to learn about these things in a more intimate setting with your lover. This is what I did, though in retrospect I think joining a class of lesbians would have been rewarding. Indeed, in some larger

Childbirth Methods

Many different methods of childbirth are taught in classes today. The most popular of them is the Lamaze method, or some derivative of Lamaze. This method acknowledges that childbirth is painful, and it focuses on natural childbirth. Lamaze emphasizes breathing to control pain, relaxing as much as possible, and being as informed as you can be in advance about the birthing process. Partners will be coached to encourage breathing and support the birthing woman through each contraction. Other methods commonly discussed in childbirth classes are the Read Method or the Bradley Method (or "husband-coached childbirth"). If you adopt a style such as this, you'll probably want to refer to it as "partner-coached."

Most sessions last about an hour and a half, and the classes extend over four to six weeks. How do you decide which method suits you best? Talk to your partner, talk to your doctor or midwife, and think about what may be the best approach for you. Find a supportive instructor who answers questions patiently and explains things clearly. And remember that once you are in labor you won't necessarily be thinking about methodology—you'll just be applying the best of what you learned to what's really happening.

---

cities you can find childbirth classes offered specifically for lesbian couples, often by an experienced lesbian midwife. If no such classes exist where you live, see if you can get one going. Ask your doctor if she will help set up such a program. Most childbirth educators can be hired for a small group of couples, and the group can meet in one couple's home.

The experience of taking birth classes as a lesbian or a lesbian couple among straight couples may initially seem intimidating. However, in most parts of North America today, most people won't bat an eye at two women attending birthing classes together. Your classmates may know or assume you're gay, or they may just think you are single and have brought along the friend who's going to be your birth coach. Or they may not think about it too much at all. After all, everyone is present at these classes for the same reason; they will all be apprehensive, excited, and focused on their own experience, just as you are. Like many aspects of pregnancy or parenting in general, birth classes may help build bridges between lesbians and straight folks.

Do Some Perineum Massage Together

Perineum massage is something you and your partner can do together in your last trimester. It's a wonderful way to prepare the perineum, the tender area between your vagina and anus, for childbirth. If you regularly massage and gently stretch out these tissues now, it may loosen the area and prevent tearing of tissue during labor. Tell your healthcare provider you're doing this massage, and see if you can plan on not having an episiotomy during labor.

To receive this massage, remove your pants and underwear and lie back on a couch or bed or on some pillows on the floor. Spread your legs, and have your partner sit between them. Relax enough so that your partner can really work the area both outside and just inside your vaginal opening. Partners, use some heated olive oil or sweet almond oil, and move your hands slowly, making gentle, firm movements. This may be uncomfortable for the pregnant woman the first few times you try it, but don't give up. Being touched in this area will feel unfamiliar to most of us, and it will require some perseverance to make this kind of touch feel routine. Eventually, you should be able to work up to a ten-minute massage every few days. You'll have tissues that are more elastic and you'll also be more aware of how to make this area expand naturally during childbirth.

Problems That Can Arise Toward the End of Pregnancy

There are no firm statistics, but it's thought that one in four pregnancies in the United States and Canada is considered high risk. High risk means that there is some danger to the mother, the baby, or both. Up to 10 percent of high-risk births are the result of labor occurring earlier than 37 weeks.

What makes a pregnancy high risk? Any of the following conditions may be evidence of something going wrong or increase the risk of complications during birth: spotting or bleeding, DES (synthetic estrogen) exposure in the woman's mother, constant or sudden high blood pressure (often called pre-eclampsia or toxemia, characterized by protein in the urine, swelling of the face and hands, and rapid weight gain), problems with the cervix or placenta (including placenta previa, where the placenta blocks the cervix, often requiring a cesarean section), and premature rupture of the amniotic sac, releasing fluid. Women expecting multiple births are often considered high risk as well. Most pregnancies involving multiples end early, and the births frequently require C-section.

You may be monitored very closely throughout your pregnancy if you have any of these conditions or are expecting multiples. You may even be prescribed bed rest during the last few weeks. This can actually make many of the discomforts of late pregnancy worse, and you may need additional help and emotional support during this time. Stay in close contact with friends, let your lover spoil you, and think about contacting a national organization called Sidelines (P.O. Box 1808, Laguna Beach, CA 92652, or www.sidelines.org), which provides support and even a buddy system for moms consigned to bed rest. The Sidelines website includes suggestions for additional reading, and they now even publish their own magazine, *Left Side Lines*.

The threat of early labor is one of the biggest hazards of late pregnancy. While your baby is no longer considered premature if it's born after 36 weeks, and not all preterm labor leads to immediate delivery, you want to keep the baby in your uterus as long as possible up to your due date. In particular, a fetus's lung development will not be optimal unless it is born close to term. If you start having contractions that persist for an hour or more, your hands and feet suddenly swell, you notice the baby moving less, you bleed from the vagina, or you suspect your water has broken, call your midwife or doctor immediately. In addition, you should let your healthcare provider know right away if you start getting severe headaches, blurred vision, abdominal or chest pains, vomiting or diarrhea, or fevers over 100 degrees.

Medical Tests You Can Expect Now

Your doctor or midwife may request frequent check-ins with you during this final stretch. Most of these appointments are just to see how you're hanging in there, and listen for the baby's heart rate. You may be tested for group B strep, and you will certainly be checked for the baby's position and "station," or how far down in your pelvis the baby has moved. If no one can tell which way the baby is lying, an ultrasound may be recommended. If the baby is in breech position, with its butt down instead of lying in a head-first position, don't panic. There are ways you can encourage the baby to turn on its own. The best way to try this is to lie with your buttocks above your head for up to twenty minutes. This may

Multiples

Mothers expecting multiple births need special care during pregnancy, and extra support after the babies arrive. While pregnant, a mom carrying multiples needs extra rest, extra protein to eat, and extra water to drink, plus special ways to get comfortable. About half of twins, and almost all triplets, are born by C-section. The risk of premature labor with twins is high, and it's especially so with triplets, with low birth weight also a frequent scenario for multiples. Because the multiples experience is largely outside the scope of this book, I urge you to seek further information elsewhere. There are several good books on pregnancy with multiples; two of the best are *When You're Expecting Twins, Triplets, or Quads: Proven Guidelines for a Healthy Multiple Pregnancy*, by Barbara Luke and Tamara Eberlein; and *The Multiple Pregnancy Sourcebook: Pregnancy and the First Days with Twins, Triplets, and More,* by Nancy Bowers.

None of these books currently includes much information on lesbian families, unfortunately. If you are expecting multiples as a lesbian parent, the Internet is an excellent source of information and networking. There are special bulletin boards created just for queer families with multiples, including one on Yahoo with 600 families on the list. A simple search of the Yahoo boards, or a Google search using keywords like "lesbian pregnancy" and "multiples," will turn these up. Also currently on Yahoo are groups for all sorts of specialized families of multiples—including parents of twin boys, special-needs twins, triplets, and even higher multiples. These boards are wonderful sources of support for expectant and new parents.

give the baby a signal it's heading in the wrong direction. You can also have your provider gently try to turn the baby by manipulating and pressing on your belly. This process is called "external version" and is worth a try. Most babies lying in breech position turn themselves before 34 weeks. If yours turns breech after this, and simply won't budge, you may need to have a C-section.

At your final appointments, your cervix will be checked for softening and to see if it has begun to open. You may be given a "nonstress test" with an external fetal monitor to measure the baby's heartbeat and movements. If there is a problem, real or perceived (the baby may just be sleeping), you may have to undergo a more invasive "stress test." It's best to have the need for these tests explained to you in advance. If you know your baby has been active in utero, usually there is no cause for either test. However, if you haven't noticed any fetal movements in a few days, tell your doctor immediately. Your doctor may even do tests to check the state of your placenta. Also in the last week or so, some caregivers "strip the membranes" by pushing away the thin skin covering the cervix. This is uncomfortable for the pregnant woman, unnecessary, and may start labor prematurely. Tell your caregiver you don't wish this done.

Will My Baby Be an Alien? and Other Normal Anxieties

In the few short weeks before the baby arrives, you'll be focusing more and more on the birth and less on the long months behind you. It's perfectly normal now to really conceptualize the size of the baby inside you and wonder how it's ever going to get out.

> I remember seeing the movies of actual births in childbirth class and thinking very strongly, with my hand on my swollen stomach, "I'm not doing that. This thing's not coming out of me that way. They'll have to think of some other way." Yeah, right! —Chris

Of course, all babies seem to get out, one way or another. You've probably had enough prenatal testing and poking and prodding from your healthcare providers to know at least the approximate size of your fetus. You probably know the baby's position and whether its head has dropped into position for birth. Therefore, you may have some idea if you're at risk for a C-section or your plans to give birth naturally are realistic. It's a good idea to finalize your hospital birth plans now, and to get everything ready if you're planning a home birth.

You may also be feeling anxiety about whether the baby is really as healthy as you've been led to believe. For example, all through my last trimester I worried about whether my baby would be normal. When people said I looked small for eight months, I'd worry that the kid would be abnormally tiny. When they said I looked huge, I worried I was going to pop a ten-pounder. My girlfriend at the time teased me by saying the baby's hiccups were actually the croaks of a giant green frog that would leap out at any moment. Far-fetched? Of course. But just the sort of comment a very pregnant woman will worry about.

> *Don't worry that your baby will turn out like an alien if you have an unknown donor. Even when they were about to do my C-section, I said to the nurse, "I'm a little worried about what this child will look like," and she told me not to worry, that he would be beautiful. And sure enough, he is. —Lillian*

What Will You Name the Baby?

Naming your baby is one of the most fun things about having one. It is also a big responsibility. Some women spend years compiling a list of favorite names. Some let their partner name the baby. Others combine the two first names or even last names of the moms into a new name for their kid. Women often name their children after a favored relative, or honor a family or religious tradition by their naming. Others make up names that are absolutely unique and previously unknown. Knowing whether you are having a boy or a girl narrows down the choices to one gender, though you should always keep a backup name of the opposite sex, in case you're surprised. If you don't know the baby's sex, you'll have to compile two lists, or choose androgynous names that can be used for either sex. Keep in mind that androgynous names once used for boys, like Jordan, often become almost exclusively girls names once the feminine usage becomes popular.

If you are single, you can pick the name or names you like without much argument from anyone. If you're partnered, you may have decided together on the perfect name already, or you might need further negotiation. Couples may find it helpful to separately compile lists of preferred names, then compare them. There may be overlap, or names that one partner finds absolutely unusable. You may like the name Lucy, for example, but your partner might have an ex-lover with a dog named Lucy. If you love a particular name so much you just can't bear not to use it, consider making it a middle name. And don't be afraid to change your ideas about names as your pregnancy progresses. Perhaps that perfect name you picked as a teenager for your future baby-to-be now sounds ridiculous, or dated. Or maybe in the meantime too many other parents discovered it too. Consult lists of popular names and try to avoid them. I remember the year the name Isabelle raged through the San Francisco parenting community. It was so common for a while I actually shuddered when introduced to the ninth or tenth baby Isabelle in a single six-month span.

There are plenty of online sites that include tips on naming, and there are numerous very inclusive baby-name books. One I liked was *The Everything Baby Names Book,* by Lisa Shaw, which comprises more than 25,000 names, including African American names and international names, including all their definitions. Try to find something unusual, or classic but underused (like Frances, for example!). Be sure the name can be spoken and spelled easily, and that it works in combination with your chosen middle and last name. Say it all aloud numerous times. Make sure it's not so long or so weird that your kid curses you later. Think about what your child's full name might be shortened to as a nickname. Confirm that your kid's initials don't spell out a profanity or anything embarrassing, like "PIG." Yes, it does happen. And no matter how spiritual or empowered you feel during your pregnancy, avoid the names of mythological gods and goddesses. I know, I love the name Artemis too, but there really should be no little babies named Demeter, Zeus, and Thor. And unless you're a celebrity, don't name your baby anything like Brooklyn or Apple.

Some names I love and hardly ever see include Felicia, Hesper ("evening star"), Marina ("from the sea"), Delilah, Zander, Gabriel, Gideon, Adam, and Jared. Feel free to use any of these—and then send me a picture of your baby!

This Woman Deserves a Party

Your Baby Shower

Most showers are given during the third trimester, and many occur in the last weeks of a pregnancy. It is traditional for a friend or relative of the pregnant woman to throw the shower, but I have heard of women giving a shower for themselves. Why not? Every pregnant woman deserves a party, and a shower is the perfect opportunity to gather together all the important people in your life and rejoice in the expected arrival of the new clan member.

Often, coworkers hold a shower for a pregnant staff person at her workplace. In that case, you would be lucky: You'd have at least two showers—one at work, and one for friends and family. Or maybe a relative wants to hold one for you—with only family members invited. And then you might have another one just for friends. That's a lot of partying—and a whole lotta gifts. I have found that most dykes, living in bigger cities with their lovers, usually just have one shower—with some family, a few coworkers, and lots of friends attending. There may even be a couple with a young child present, letting you know what you're in for. Showers can also be a time, especially for single mamas, to get a sense of commitment from friends to care for you and the baby in the immediate weeks (and ideally, months) after the baby's birth. You may want to put it out there that the best gift you could receive is the knowledge that your friends won't all disappear after the baby comes home!

Some people think that only women should attend a shower, but feel free to invite whomever you want, without relying on old, outdated traditions. The age of the co-ed queer baby shower is definitely here.

What happens at a baby shower? There are entire books dedicated to the "proper" way to hold one, including how to send invitations, decorate, choose food, and plan games and activities. This seemed completely overwhelming for me to consider while pregnant, so thank goodness I had a friend who volunteered to host mine. There was a yummy "Happy Baby" cake, finger food, and nonalcoholic drinks. I considered most of the traditional baby shower games so ridiculous for my circle of hip urban dyke friends that I vetoed them all. Instead, I used the time to mix with and enjoy the company of my friends, many of whom I hadn't seen much during my pregnancy. There was lots of food and good conversation, and the party had none of the stress that might accompany a more organized affair!

Typically, showers are a way, especially for first-time moms, to receive often expensive goodies for the baby from generous friends. But if you're in the loop of hand-me-downs as I was, there's little you'll really need by the time the shower rolls around. Instead, concentrate on the celebratory nature of the day and revel in being the center of attention one last time—next time there's a large gathering, the baby will steal the show!

Shower invitations should be sent out several weeks in advance; list the time and place, as well as the host's name and phone number. Encourage people to RSVP so the host will know how much food to buy and prepare. Saturday or Sunday afternoons are good times for many people. If you are using a registry, include that information on your invites. Some stores use electronic wands to scan items and automatically add, and then subtract, these items from a wish-list. Although some people consider any specific requests rude, I think it is better to let folks know if there are items you really need—or don't. For example, because I had already received several boxes of infant and baby clothes by the time shower day came around, I indicated that people should not buy any clothes smaller than one-year size. I couldn't bear to think of my friends wasting their money on items I would never use because I already had a surplus.

While few people can resist buying one or two teeny-weeny outfits for you, there are other more practical items you can express interest in, and many are almost cost-free. If people ask, here are some suggestions you'll be happy to have made:

Noncommercial Gifts That Will Ring Mom's Bell

- Shopping and cooking dinner for Mom during the baby's first month home. This is a particularly perfect gift for the single mama!
- Cleaning Mom's bathroom for about two weeks after the baby's born. This is a time when you can't bend over, you're still bleeding all over everything, and dirt anywhere will be bothersome. Oh, how I wished someone had offered to do this for me, but I was too embarrassed to ask. Eventually, I hired someone to come in and clean for me a few times, mostly to give my bathroom a good scrub.
- Coming over to play with the baby while Mom takes a good long bath—or nap
- A gift certificate for an at-home massage or a dinner delivery
- An offer to take photos of Mom(s) and baby, complete with developing double sets of photos

Gifts to request of people who want to buy substantial store-bought presents include a baby carrier like a front pack or a sling, a new car seat, a good quality diaper bag, or a vibrating bouncy seat or baby swing.

After the shower, send out thank-you notes almost immediately, so that the task isn't hanging over your head in the short weeks before labor. You never know when Junior might make an early arrival!

Further Preparations

Other Stuff to Have Around Before the Birth

- Maximum-size sanitary pads for postbirth discharge (known as lochia) and bleeding. You will need these unless you have a planned C-section. And yes, get the maximum size.
- Breast pads in case you leak a lot
- A few packs of diapers—but not all in newborn size, as the baby will outgrow these very quickly
- Rubbing alcohol and Q-Tips to clean the baby's umbilical stump
- Diaper rash cream, or a "natural" equivalent like Burt's Bees "Baby Bee Cream"
- Very mild baby soap and baby lotion
- Baby-sized nail clippers—the baby's nails will be long and sharp!
- Bottles and formula if you plan to bottle-feed
- Frozen food and bottled juice and water, for you
- Book on newborn care (I can take you only so far!)
- A battery-operated vibrating bouncy chair—a place to actually put a baby down when you need to go pee or just need a break. Also great for soothing fussy babies. Mine absolutely loved it.

What Is a Receiving Blanket, Anyway?

I figure the term must come from the fact that you "receive" the baby wrapped up in one of these, but who knows what its exact origin is. In any case, receiving blankets are those tiny blankets of cotton or other soft, breathable material that you will use to wrap the baby in, especially when they are newborn or you go outside. Receiving blankets keep the baby warm and are easier to use than putting multiple layers of clothing on a tiny, squirming baby. They are portable and easily stored in different rooms of the house or in the car for quick access. Swaddle your newborn in one during its first few days at home; your baby will find this very comforting. You will probably get a few receiving blankets as presents; if not, go buy a few. You can use them for blankets in the baby's crib later on.

Packing It Up

Even if you are planning a home birth, it's a good idea to pack a hospital bag containing both necessities and items that will make your possible hospital stay more comfortable. My advice is to have this ready about a month early, so that you don't leave it to chance in a possibly sudden departure to the hospital. Don't forget to have a plan ready for other children in the family, and make preparations for pet care.

What to Pack for Delivery

FOR THE BIRTHING MOM

- Nightgown or comfortable, loose sleeping wear
- Warm socks or polar fleece slippers to protect your feet against cold hospital floors
- Bras (if you wear them) or a nursing bra
- Heavy-duty maxi pads for postdelivery bleeding
- Several packs of your favorite, small-sized hard candies to suck on during delivery
- Eyeglasses, especially if you normally wear contacts
- Lip balm
- Your own shampoo and soap, and a soft towel
- Trashy mags or a book, in case you need to stay a while
- A clean outfit to wear home
- Any insurance papers you may need
- Essential oils, like lavender, that you may wish to use
- Candles and matches

FOR THE OTHER MOM OR BIRTHING PARTNER

- Massage oil
- Cassette or CD player if you want to play music (make sure batteries are working and music is loaded!)
- Camera or video with film already loaded and working batteries
- Coins for the pay phone and the list of phone numbers to call. If you have one, your cell phone and its charger
- Snacks and bottled water or other hydrating drinks
- A change of clothes
- A swimsuit, in case your partner wants you with her in the shower and you're not the type to get bare naked in front of a bunch of other folks

FOR THE BABY

- A name—since most hospitals won't discharge you without a name on the birth certificate
- A receiving blanket
- Newborn-sized diapers
- A newborn-sized outfit to wear home, complete with a hat to keep the baby's head warm
- A rear-facing infant car seat, as is the law in all 50 states
- Your "baby book," if you want a handprint or footprint officially recorded at the hospital

If You Are Planning a Home Birth

If you are preparing to give birth at home, your midwife will have you order a recommended "birth kit." These are commercially prepared for home births and contain necessary items such as a plastic sheet for the birthing area, underpads, gauze, special homeopathic drugs like arnica pills (200c) to heal postbirth bruising and soreness, and a sitz bath. The kits also include items necessary for the baby such as a bulb syringe and newborn stocking caps. In addition, you will need to have extra towels and plastic tarps, sanitary napkins, and cleaning items such as bleach on hand. Have everything prepared according to the midwife's instructions, and keep her phone number with you wherever you go during these last few weeks.

It's also advisable to stock up on items like juice, ice, coffee, clear soups, and prepackaged snacks for those attending the birth. Labor can sometimes take a few days, and three o'clock in the morning is not the time to realize that there's no food in the house.

Make sure you have your phone list beside the telephone, all your sheets and towels clean (you'll go through a ton in the first few days), and know how to register your baby's birth in your particular city or town. You may need the midwife to sign papers or fill out a mock birth certificate at the time of the baby's arrival. Better to know exactly what you need before you schlep down to City Hall with the new baby in tow.

The Circumcision Decision

Without the pressure to have a baby boy "look just like Dad," I believe lesbians should have greater clarity than straight folks on the circumcision issue. Yet while we abhor the practice of female circumcision in developing countries, we remain largely ignorant of the practice we willingly perform on our own sons. I personally find this inexcusable. Circumcision is a largely unnecessary medical procedure that causes an infant great pain. Yet, large numbers of lesbians still have their sons circumcised, some for religious reasons, but many because they are just following what they think is "normal" procedure. But if we are ever going to demand that society change its perceptions about what is normal, we should also look at the larger issues of childrearing and consider how we can change them.

Male circumcision, which is performed on about 60 percent of American baby boys (but only about 20 percent of baby boys worldwide), is the surgical removal of the foreskin of a boy's penis. It is usually performed without anesthetic, even in hospitals, so the baby must be strapped down to a board or table. They cry so hard they can barely breathe.

There used to be speculation that circumcision might prevent infections and penile cancer later in a boy's life, but the rates of these ailments are very low, and any boy can easily be taught how to care for himself and stay clean. It was also popularized as a means to keep young boys from masturbating, and that certainly has never worked. Most childbirth educators and pregnancy book authors, as well as the American Academy of Pediatrics, no longer recommend circumcision. Babies feel pain, and I don't believe parents should subject a trusting young infant to this kind of trauma. Please think carefully about this issue before deciding to simply follow in someone else's footsteps.

If you are Jewish and feel that circumcision is an important part of your cultural heritage, consider substituting some other ritual for the *bris*. Many such ceremonies now emphasize the cutting of an item other than the infant's body, and the event becomes a "naming ceremony" rather than a surgery. This type of alternative ceremony can be held for a boy or a girl child. Listed below are the websites of several organizations offering information on circumcision and alternative ceremonies.

- A direct link to a site that features an alternative *bris*, called a *bris shalom*, that does no harm:
  www.cirp.org/pages/cultural/bris_shalom.html
- No Harm (National Organization to Halt the Abuse and Routine Mutilation of Males): www.noharmm.org
- National Organization of Circumcision Information Resource Centers: www.nocirc.org

Lest you think I am being too harsh, this is what trusted childbirth educator Sheila Kitzinger has written about circumcision in her classic *The Complete Book of Pregnancy and Childbirth*: "Whether a baby cries or is overwhelmed by shock, he has a raw and painful scar afterwards.... Sometimes a mother observes her baby's personality seems to have changed. The rhythms of love between a mother and her newborn are disrupted. We can only guess the possible long-term emotional effects of this mutilating surgery."

By the way, female genital mutilation is now a felony in the United States. Perhaps, one day, male circumcision will be too.

Last-Minute Legal Advice

If you haven't already followed up on some of the legal advice I've given you in this book, now is the time to do so. Although some legal agreements (like a second-parent adoption) cannot be completed until the baby is born, one thing you can do now is make sure you have a valid will. Many people never make a will; but now that you are on the verge of parenthood, be a grown-up and get one done! Particularly since the law does not protect lesbians very well, a will can provide substantial proof of who and what is important in your life. It's always best to see a lawyer, but Nolo Press has published some good books on writing your own will, with forms provided.

> Before the baby arrives, have a will drawn up as well as any other necessary legal documents. I know that I had this huge fear of "What if something happens to me while I am giving birth?" I had already made my wishes clear to my mother and to anyone who would listen that if anything ever happened to me, the baby should be with my partner. But in a time of loss and crisis, I'm not sure what steps my Mom would take, even though she promised. I strongly recommend seeing a lawyer and making sure everything is taken care of, just in case. —Mona

Surviving Those Last Few Weeks

> I think the purpose of the last month is to convince every cell of your being that you are ready for the next stage, even if it does

mean labor and delivery of unknown type and duration, only to be followed by a little person for whom you have no idea how to care. —Jen

Ugh. My last few weeks were entirely uncomfortable. Most women who carry to full term or beyond find the last month a really difficult time. Not only does the baby go through a growth spurt in the last month, but it will also stay really active. Sleeping becomes very difficult for the birthing mom, it's hard to get comfortable enough to sleep, and you may wake up many times a night to pee. You will probably be tired a lot.

My last month was miserable. I was huge, and the baby kept bouncing on a nerve at the bottom of my spine, which would cause me to yelp in pain at the oddest times. I peed constantly and lumbered everywhere. My mantra for the last trimester was "I bend for no one." As for sleep...forget it! Didn't do it much for the first six months afterward anyway—maybe that last month was simply prep work for what was to come. —Jody

This is also a tough time emotionally. You are so ready to meet your baby, and so over being pregnant. And you may be emotionally on edge. I was sick of answering questions about my very public pregnancy, and I thought some days that if I heard the questions "Do you know if it's a boy or a girl?" and "Are you excited?" one more time I might very well lose it. Part of this was probably caused by lack of sleep, part by physical discomfort, and part by real impatience to put these ten months of pregnancy behind me. I was impatient for something—anything—to happen.

Finding time to be alone, or just with your partner, may become more important during the last few weeks of your pregnancy. I had a sudden realization that these were my last few days to ever really spend alone, and I cherished the little bits of solitude I could carve out for myself. Whatever else is going on, try to escape from people a bit if you can—go sit in the park, or have a bath. There's nothing quite like lighting some candles, shutting the bathroom door, and escaping into a bubble bath.

At the same time you find you need solitude, you'll also notice things starting to get very busy. People begin calling every day to see how you are, relatives may start arriving to stay with you, and last-minute preparations for the baby are in full swing. Suddenly, you can become very busy just when you need to rest. It's important to stay calm and claim this time as your own, no matter how you choose to spend it. If you have a partner, try to enjoy this last bit of couple time by going out for a special meal or treating each other to a massage. The more connected you feel to each other emotionally before going into labor, the better.

If you are sexually intimate these last few weeks, you may notice it's harder to get into a comfortable position. You may experience some contractions after orgasm, and your breasts may leak a bit. These are normal occurrences, and they will not make you go into labor unless your baby is ready to be born. However, nipple stimulation does release oxytocin, a hormone that stimulates milk production (and that can be given in chemical form during labor to keep things progressing). So don't do any nipple play unless you're really ready for the baby's arrival!

And though it may be hard, try to exercise. If you haven't had previous complications, a little exercise will keep you limber for the work of labor. While you're exercising, don't wear anything too tight, and don't do any sit-ups, lunges, or anything that can stress your already strained ligaments. Swimming, stretching, squatting, and walking are good. If it's hot, go walk around an air-conditioned mall. Practice your breathing exercises as you walk. If you're still at work, carry a bag of healthy snacks and water with you, and put your feet up whenever you can.

"False" Labor and "Overdue" Babies

You may experience symptoms referred to as false labor—or practice labor—anytime close to your due date. Practice labor's contractions are sporadic, only mildly strong without gaining in intensity, and they usually stop if you change positions. I prefer the term *practice labor* to the more common medical usage *false labor*. Calling something "false" carries a negative connotation, and it can be used derisively against many first-time moms who have no way of knowing if this is really it. Certainly, if you think you're in labor, get checked by your midwife or doctor. If you arrive at the hospital thinking your labor has started, only to be sent home again, it can be very disappointing. Try to rest, continue to eat normally, and know that "real" labor will come soon. After a touch of practice labor, you'll notice a marked difference in how real labor feels.

What does "overdue" mean? Usually, when a woman goes past her due date, she is considered overdue. Since lesbians usually know to the day when they conceived, recheck your dates to ensure your due date is correctly calculated. And remember that due dates are just a guide. Rarely do first-time moms go into labor on their due dates. Unless you have been diagnosed with gestational diabetes and your baby is growing too large, it's always better to give birth a few days late than too early. Medical experts disagree on how long the baby should "bake," but midwives seldom become concerned by an extra week or ten days in the oven. Past two weeks, you will get pressure to be induced, as the baby could suffer at this point.

The Bitter End

Your pregnancy may have reached a point where you feel it is never going to end. You are at the bitter end now, but if you can just hang onto your sense of humor for a few more days, it will all be over soon! The day before my baby was due, I was feeling really cranky when I ran into an acquaintance on the street. She told me the best ways to survive the last few days of a pregnancy are to drink lots of water, walk every day, and rent funny movies. I promptly went for a long walk through the park, and then stopped by the video store and rented *GI Jane* and *Romy and Michelle's High School Reunion.* I rightly figured watching Demi Moore go through rigorous military training would make me realize that someone could indeed have it worse than I did at that moment. By the time I popped in the second film, about two silly friends who attend a school reunion, I had lightened up, and I laughed all the way through it. That was definitely some of the best advice I'd received during my pregnancy!

As your due date nears, you'll wonder how you'll recognize the signs of impending labor, and what to do if all signs are go. Turn the page to the next chapter, and I'll fill you in!

11

Birth—the Big Event

The Big Event Draws Near

The last few weeks have been hard. You've grown as big as a house, you have to pee all the time, you have heartburn, your ligaments hurt, and you can't sleep. You are probably asking yourself when this whole thing is going to be over. Most likely you've stopped thinking of all those months you spent inseminating, and you can't imagine yourself not pregnant. Part of you is desperate to get this baby out. Another part can't imagine how it's going to get out.

Emotionally, you might find this a hard time. So much of the last few weeks seems to be about waiting. Friends and family are tired of asking how you are and are now just waiting for your big news. Your partner may be impatient with your pregnancy and anxiously waiting to jump in as a full-fledged parent. And you're getting crabby waiting for this baby to come. Really, really, crabby.

Luckily, by the time you're feeling the most fed up, your body is already preparing for childbirth. Many women are worried about how they will know labor has begun. How can you tell your labor is beginning? My mother said she could tell my labor had begun because I suddenly was very restless and irritable. Here are some other, more medically proven, clues.

Is It Really Time? Some Surefire Signs

One of the first signs that labor may soon begin is called lightening, and it means the baby has dropped down deep and low in your pelvis. People may look at you and be able to tell this has happened even if you don't feel it. Your vagina may feel bigger and softer. Or your midwife may notice changes in your cervix as it softens and ripens for the baby's passage through. When I was checked a few days before labor kicked in, we found my cervix had moved down and was extremely soft, spongy, and flat. I had already dilated enough so that a finger could be inserted through the opening. It's normal to dilate a centimeter or two before real labor begins, and your doctor or midwife will be checking for this. In fact, you could be 1 or 2 centimeters dilated for a week or more. It's a surefire sign your labor is in its beginning stage.

Another sign of impending labor is the beginning of persistent Braxton-Hicks contractions. You may feel these for months before your due date, but now you might notice them more and more frequently. Your abdomen may feel incredibly hard when these contractions hit, almost as if you could bounce a ball off your tummy. Other signs include backache, weird cramps that make you feel as though you're about to get your period, an upset stomach, and even vomiting. When it comes right down to it, though, there are three surefire ways to tell if labor has really begun: passing the mucus plug, having your bag of waters break, and feeling the onslaught of real contractions. Unfortunately, not every woman experiences the first two, so you may be hot with contractions before you realize that things are really under way.

It can be hard to think of anything but your own discomfort now. Having been there, I know this discomfort is real. But remember how lucky you are. Know that other women are looking at you as a role model, many with envy in their eyes.

Passing the Mucus Plug

During my entire pregnancy, my girlfriend at the time and I joked about the moment when the mucus plug would come hurtling out of me. Of course, this was a gross exaggeration of what we knew would happen, but we liked to kid around about it. The mucus plug is a gelatinous separator between the cervix and the uterus; its appearance may mean labor is coming, because when the cervix starts to widen the plug will come out. However, some women pass this plug— also called *bloody show*—weeks before their labor starts, and others never see it, since it simply gets lost in the messiness of labor itself. Right when I was wondering whether my labor was starting, I went to the bathroom to pee and found that the toilet tissue was full of thick mucus that looked a lot like bloody spin. It was the indicator I'd been looking for, and seeing the plug was a reassuring—and a terrifying—moment. Labor had begun!

The Waters Run Wide

Many women at this stage are anxiously wondering how and when their waters will break. Will it be at night, thereby soaking the bed? Or in the health-food store, in the crowded produce aisle? Or in the park, with small children gaping? There's certainly no way to know when and where, or even if indeed your waters will actually break. Women giving birth in the hospital have their waters broken to induce labor, while babies born at home are sometimes delivered right in their sacs.

What does it actually mean that your waters break? You already know that the baby has been kept safe in an amniotic sac inside your body throughout your entire pregnancy. When it's time for labor to begin, the sac often breaks.

Despite the fact that we are trained by popular culture to view the breaking of the waters as a surefire, commonplace sign that the baby's coming, in reality, only a small percentage of women experience this in a dramatic fashion. In fact, fewer than 10 percent of women have their waters break before labor. If all you know of labor is what you see on TV shows and movies, you'd expect to see a huge gush of water, and then a woman lying on her back in a hospital bed for a few hours, and then a baby pulled out while she screams. This is not reality, gals, so try not to impose any of that model on yourself or your partner.

If you are worried about your waters breaking while you sleep, you can place plastic sheets or towels on your bed. If you're really concerned, you could always wear a sanitary pad during your last week or two. I decided to take my chances, and as it turned out, the midwives elected to break my waters when I was already well into labor. Not because they absolutely had to, mind you, but because my labor had stalled and it was one of their tricks to help things along.

If you're still worried, know that many women's waters do not break until contractions are well under way, in which case you'll probably be safely at home or in the hospital anyway. It may come out in a sudden rush or trickle out, depending on whether the baby's head is blocking the flow of water. If your waters break and labor does not progress, your caregiver probably has strong views about how long you can go before recommending intervention. If your waters break and labor hasn't begun within the next twelve hours, your labor will likely be induced. This is a topic that experts differ about, so it is best to know your caregiver's philosophy about this in advance.

When your waters do break, check the color of the fluid itself. If it's got traces of brown or green in it, rather than appearing clear, it may contain meconium (your baby's first poop). It is actually harmful for your baby to be exposed to this in utero, and could indicate fetal distress. Your provider will need to know right away if this is the case.

Most women go into labor in the evening hours, and most babies are born at night. Legend has it that this is because in prehistoric times predators could see and therefore prey on newborn infants born in daylight. If it was dark, infants had a better chance of surviving till morning. Many people also believe more babies are born on the full moon.

The Contractions Begin

A typical labor may begin with contractions that come about ten to 20 minutes apart, and last 30 seconds to a minute. They will get longer and stronger and eventually come about every two to five minutes, until you hit transition. More on contractions and the different stages of labor in upcoming sections. Every woman's contractions are different; you'll know them when they start coming. Some birth writers call contractions "expansions," or even "rushes," to try to empower women with more positive imagery of labor. Whatever you call them, the pain of the contractions will make you feel as though your entire insides are shuddering.

Most pregnancy books state that contractions start far apart, and when they are close together the baby is about to come. I've heard of women who do things like bake a cake between contractions. Ha! In my labor, the contractions started pretty close together, and there was never much of a break in between. I could barely walk from the bedroom to the bathroom without having a contraction on the way there, and then another while I was on the toilet. Which, by the way, is a great place to spend some time during late labor, as it is almost a perfect birthing chair!

The Excitement of It All

A Time Like No Other

Labor is a time like no other. All your regular perceptions about time and space and your physical being are thrown to the wind. A measured hour means nothing. Some moments during labor feel like hours, especially when you are having a contraction, yet the hours slip away into a haze of passing time. Make sure that when labor starts you are safely where you need to be—at home, a birthing room, or the hospital. Once your contractions get intense, it will be very difficult to move to another location. With my partner's assistance, I had to walk from her house to my own during early labor—a distance of only a few blocks. It was a seemingly unending journey, taking a few steps at a time between contractions. When a contraction arrived, I clutched at poles and fire hydrants and even my partner, aware that my odd behavior was eliciting stares from strangers. Those scenes in films—with the woman inside a cab, breathing hard, eyes scrunched up and clutching her tummy—do not show you the overwhelming physical sensations she would really be having.

As soon as you know your labor is happening, get grounded. Be where you need to be, have all your supplies at hand, make sure you have food for the next few days at the ready, and a list of people to call by the phone. Make sure the pets are accounted for and walked or fed, or given to a friend for a day or two. Pick up the other kids from school, and promptly put your plan for them into action. If the children are going to be part of the birth experience, make sure their adult birth companion is on-notice or coming right over. If the children are to be taken to a relative or a friends' home, make sure a bag has been packed for their time away—including a beloved blanket or stuffed animal that can help during the separation.

Then prepare yourself to be swept away in the unbelievable experience that is about to begin.

Imagine a Natural Birth

When I say to prepare to be swept away, I am not advising you let go of the kind of birth you want. I'm only letting you in on the fact that you won't be able to control everything that happens to you in your birth journey. This can be hard to understand, since the clearer you are about your birth choices in advance, the more they will be actualized. It is easy to see how a first-time pregnant mom could be inundated with birth horror stories and relatives who pressure her to have a "safe" birth in the hospital. The women I know who've had the most medical intervention when they gave birth are medical doctors. Why might this be? Probably because they have too much faith in medical intervention and not enough in the amazing capabilities of the healthy human body. Med school probably taught them not to rely on the powers of their own body to birth a baby. In fact, one doctor I know, a confident and successful woman, had an emergency cesarean experience so horrific that the story made me shudder for weeks afterward.

By deciding on a home birth without pain medicine, I issued myself a challenge. This challenge was to reject the medical model of childbirth, to summon all the strength I knew I possessed as a woman, and let the experienced hands of my midwives guide me along my birth journey. I also was concerned that one intervention would lead to another, and I would have the disassociated medical birth my mother had had with me. Concerns that my child not be born with any drugs in her system also motivated me to keep my birth drug-free. I still feel incredibly empowered by having made these choices, and by having a home birth. Can you allow yourself to imagine this kind of experience? Read the holistic *Birthing From Within*, by Pam England, and any writing on childbirth by Ina May Gaskin for more inspiration on this topic.

Let Your Partner Share the Experience

If you have a partner, you'll be counting on her to be steady for you during labor. But allow her to be swept away in this amazing experience, too. Having a supportive doula, midwife, friend, or family member present can take some of the burden off your partner to be "perfect" during your labor. This person can also help deal with hospital staff or with situations that might take your partner away from your side, like running out to get a snack for you or making some phone calls. Especially helpful will be a female friend or family member who has been though or witnessed natural childbirth before. Remember—birth is a transformative experience for the nonbirthing partner, too.

Don't Make Promises

That said, it's best to make no promises to anyone about attending your labor. I told two of my best friends, one of them the photographer who was supposed to take pictures of my baby's birth, that I would call them as soon as I went into labor. That never happened. I felt weird about calling them late at night when my labor was confirmed, and by the time morning rolled around, I was no longer thinking rationally about anything. My entire being was focused on the journey my baby and I were catapulting our way along on, and I could barely remember my name, let alone the friends I had promised to call. The midwives, my mother, my partner at the time, and I had operated as a small, well-coordinated birth team for more than 12 hours already, and bringing anyone else into the equation would have felt wrong, especially in my tiny apartment. Labor is just too intense and surreal an experience to know how you're going to feel ahead of time. Of course, my friends were very disappointed. But it's your birth experience, so do what you need to do, and don't feel guilty about it.

What Is Labor Like?

Each woman has a completely different experience during labor. Hearing stories of easy deliveries (like "it was only three hours long and I hardly had to push at all") and thinking that you will have a quick, easy labor will most likely lead to disappointment. Don't be scared by the horror stories you've heard, even if most of them are true. Some birth educators believe that a woman's first birth is usually similar to those of her mother and sisters. That being said, your birth will be your very own.

There are books full of birthing stories in print, but after reading a few of these collections, I feel certain voices were missing. Certainly, there are fewer stories of home births than hospital births, and almost no stories from lesbian moms. That is why I am so glad that more lesbian writers are publishing first-person accounts of their pregnancies and births. Here are a few special tidbits from lesbian moms about their labors:

> *The pain didn't matter anymore, it was just everywhere and always. The last part of labor hurt me the most, because the crowning "ring of fire" is no exaggeration term! But some part of me was still coherent and listened when the midwife said, "Don't push anymore, breathe it out." I did breathe and after only a few more contractions suddenly I felt a big warm gush and then a squirmy wet thing was in my lap! I remember saying several times "I'm so glad it's over!" and crying before I realized the little squirmy thing was my baby. —Tamara*

> *Because of the epidural, I gave birth on the hospital bed. My partner, Julie, held my left leg, and a nurse held my right leg, and as I pushed against both of them, our daughter, Ani, began to come into the world. With my first push there was a lot of excitement and activity, because Ani's head had crowned. She was all the way down the birth canal and just waiting for me to take her the rest of the way. Every time I pushed, you could see a little more of her head, and when I took a break, her head receded. They set up a full-length mirror so I could watch myself deliver, and it was the most amazing experience of my life, watching myself push and seeing her head come out more and more. We were chanting, "Come on baby, come on baby, we can do it, come on baby." And all of a sudden, literally, out popped her little head! Dark hair, round little face all scrunched up, the rest of her body still inside me. I heard Julie say, "She's here!" and no sooner had she said it than Ani turned her head toward Julie and opened her eyes to look right at her. It was unbelievable to realize that she recognized Julie's voice. We were both crying with awe and amazement! —Catherine*

I'm a single mom and had my best (male) friend as my coach. Wasn't it a hoot when he got to wear the "father" wristband! My labor was quick—just about four hours from start to finish. Hardly time to get settled in and get used to it. I kept my eyes closed during most of it so I could focus, but I'd look up and make sure my coach was there. I hadn't realized how much I'd need that comfort. —Stella

My labor room at the hospital looked out over a eucalyptus tree grove. I found myself swaying back and forth through my contractions, in time to the eucalyptus trees. —Ingrid

My first baby was born in a hospital. Although everything went well, I knew I wanted to have a home birth with my second child. In fact, I not only had a home birth but had a water birth. I rented a birth tank and found myself actually looking forward to labor to try it out! This time the birth was much easier, in part because I knew what I was doing and what I wanted. My partner was naked and in the water much of the time with me. Although the baby was actually born out of the water, the tank really helped me with the most painful parts of labor. The whole experience was altogether amazing! —Jennifer

All the scariness melted away as soon as my midwife arrived and I felt like someone was there to support me. I found the contractions manageable and even though pushing the baby out hurt, it was an unbelievable feeling to finally welcome him into the world. —Mai

Remember that the baby is in labor with you. Inside your body, he or she is surging with catecholamine hormones, ready to do the work of being born. You need not worry about the baby suffering in a normal vaginal birth, for though it feels the contractions squeeze and push, he or she is well equipped for this journey. Once out in the world, babies that are vaginally born, especially without drugs, are usually alert and calm. They are ready to see the face of the most important person in the world—the one who just gave birth. Keep the lights dim and your baby close. This is a magical moment.

The Three Stages of Labor

Three stages of labor are common to every natural birth. A very simple way to think of these stages is that the first involves the body preparing itself for the baby's birth, the second involves getting the baby out, and the last involves birthing the placenta. The clinical terms for these stages are:

- Stage 1: Early Labor, Active Labor, and Transition
- Stage 2: Birth
- Stage 3: Afterbirth—Birthing the Placenta

If you have a hospital birth, you may be told you're in a certain "phase" of labor. In a home birth, the stages will likely all flow into one another. While I think it's useful to know the stages of labor, I recommend not placing too much import on where you are in this journey. It will happen in its own time, in its own way. It may be good to know that the discomfort of transition will be passing soon, or that it's almost time to push. But don't feel you have to remember all these steps while you're in labor. Your midwife or nurse can advise you along the way if there is a reason to know what stage you're in.

Here is a quick overview of each phase.

Stage 1: Early Labor, Active Labor, and Transition

EARLY LABOR

Many books advise trying to ignore early labor. I suppose if it's your second baby, and you know what to expect, you might be able to watch some TV or play a game of cards, but I found this impossible. How could I ignore throwing up while violent waves of nausea passed over me? Or ignore my body trembling with pain? Or the anxiety and excitement I felt, beginning at 10 P.M., when I realized my labor was actually starting? If this is your first baby, you probably won't be able to ignore early labor either. You can try to do the things people suggest for distraction, such as going to a movie, having a bath, or taking a walk. But my bet is, if you're like me and your contractions start with a bang, early labor cannot be ignored. You'll want to be safely home or on your way to the hospital so you can hunker down for what's to come.

During early labor, many women think they have dilated farther than they have, and they go to the hospital only to be sent home till the next day. While this is very disappointing, and you won't want to leave, try to relax at home for at least a few hours till you head back to the hospital. If you're having a home birth, call your midwife now to let her know you think your labor has started. If your contractions have just started, she may not want to come over yet, but you can ask her to come check you if possible. When I first called my midwife, she doubted that I was in labor and told me to call her back in several hours. In the meantime, she told me, relax. I paced the apartment like a wild animal for several hours and then decided a bath might help me relax. I got into the tub and immediately threw up everywhere. When I called the midwife again, at around 1 A.M., she heard the hysterical note in my voice and decided to come over. As it turned out, I was already 3 centimeters dilated and my early labor was well underway.

Early labor usually lasts from six to 12 hours for first-time moms. During this time, the cervix is drawn up into the uterus, dilates (opens), and effaces (thins out). You will become increasingly agitated and uncomfortable; you may throw up and even have diarrhea. This is your body's way of purging itself to prepare for the baby's birth. All these things may happen during the course of several days, or just several hours. If you are checked multiple times during this process, you may be told that you are just 1 or 2 centimeters dilated. This can feel discouraging, since you are already primed for action. Have patience. If you're having a hospital birth, this is the time to shower and eat—you may not be allowed to do either later. Once you reach 3 centimeters, your labor will start accelerating.

ACTIVE LABOR

The phase of active labor is when things really start to happen. This is when the cervix dilates from 3 to 8 centimeters. You could be in active labor for an hour (if you've had kids before) to eight hours (which is what a lot of the books say) to 14 hours (which is about how long mine was), and there's no way to predict this in advance. The best thing you can do is pace yourself and settle in to this middle phase of labor. A hot shower may feel really good, and you can ask your partner to join you in the water. I took a long shower in midlabor that helped both calm and reinvigorate me.

You may also find you're hungry right about now. If you're at home, you can eat. If you're at the hospital, you may be placed on an IV drip, which will deliver glucose to your system. You will probably not be allowed to eat much while on the IV; in case you need a cesarean, they want your stomach empty. Although I did not want to eat much during my labor, my midwife gave me ginger ale from a spoon to hydrate me and settle my stomach, and I snacked on bits of fresh watermelon. During active labor, your contractions are coming two to five minutes apart and lasting about a minute. They may reach a peak in the middle that is most painful. Mine were so bad that I had to hang on to my partner's neck, arms wrapped around her shoulders, head pressed against her chest. Just having someone's hands on me made the contractions bearable, and the almost constant back rubbing I received was a lifesaver. You might find, on the other hand, that you don't wish to be touched at all.

The pain of contractions is not easily describable. It's not like breaking your arm or stubbing your toe. It's not really like bad menstrual cramps, either. It's a lot more constant and intense, and it comes from a place deep inside you. One friend told me she felt as if she was wracked with bad food poisoning. The pain and discomfort can easily overtake your entire being, making it hard to think clearly and be fully present. It can seem as if this pain is all you have ever known and all you will ever know.

That being said, I can also honestly tell you that the pain of labor is a manageable pain. It is nothing to run away from. It is, as my midwife says, "pain with a purpose." This purpose is to move the baby, during contractions, down through the birth canal. When you feel labor pain, your uterus, the largest muscle in your body, is squeezing tight. Your cervix is stretching as it dilates. The baby is moving through your body on its way out. Not only does all this hurt, these are not types of pain we are used to experiencing. But remember to breathe as you've been taught in childbirth classes, do your visualizing, and try guttural moaning or anything else that keeps you focused. Let your partner or labor coach know what they can do to make you more comfortable.

Moving around may feel better than trying to lie still on a bed. I found that walking around my kitchen was a good distraction. When a contraction hit, I'd drape myself over the dining-room table and put my head down on it for a moment. I didn't stay in one position very long. You should follow your body's lead and allow it to move as it wants to; don't feel you have to lie still. Usually women know instinctually how to assume positions that facilitate labor, such as walking around a bit, squatting, or even kneeling.

Active labor may tire you out the most. It seems as though you are dealing with contractions for hours and hours—and you are. It may feel as though it's all you can do to get through each contraction. That's true, too. You may start forgetting about the people around you and really begin focusing on your body.

If you're in the hospital and considering pain relief, now would be the time to ask for it. Keep in mind, though, that once you have an epidural (a shot in the spinal column that numbs your entire lower body), natural childbirth goes out the window. If you do have an epidural, you may also need to be given Pitocin (synthetic oxytocin) to stimulate labor. Then you will be hooked up to a fetal monitor. You will be flat on your back, you won't be able to move around at all, and you will no longer be as active a participant in your own baby's birth. Some circumstances call for medical intervention, of course—for example, if the mother's failure to progress in labor endangers the baby. But I would urge any of you who are considering a "routine" epidural to reconsider—and put trust in yourself and your body instead. You've managed to grow this amazing life inside you for nine months. Your body is likely also capable of giving birth to the baby just fine.

TRANSITION

Okay, the transition time is tough. You may be in a lot of pain. You may bleed a bit. You may not believe that labor can hurt this much. Your cervix is dilating from 8 to 10 centimeters to accommodate the baby's head through the birth canal, and the baby is shifting slightly sideways into the birthing position. You can feel your baby down very low and you really want to push, but it isn't time yet. I don't remember transition per se, but at a certain point when I thought, *I don't know if I can take this much longer*, my midwives told me that I was already past transition, so I knew I could take it. Transition lasts about an hour for most women, though it may feel indeterminable.

Many women get symptoms in transition like shaky legs, feelings of icy coldness or sweatiness, nausea, and irritability. And who could blame us for being irritable? Transition is really tough. This may be when you start to lose it, to disappear inside yourself, into a very alternate reality. Your voice may change from moans to grunts. You may yell at everyone around you, and lots of straight women curse at their husbands during transition for getting them pregnant. Of course, we dykes can't blame anyone except ourselves for being pregnant, so we can't do that! At this stage, lots of gals decide that they've had enough of all this pregnancy business and that they don't want a baby after all. I do have a distinct memory of squatting through a contraction and saying, "I don't want to do this anymore." Of course, there wasn't much choice about it, and it was soon time to push.

Transition can last from a few minutes to an hour or more, depending in part on the position of the baby. Contractions during transition last about a minute, and can come less than a minute apart. It's very intense, but you'll soon be able to push, and the worst will be over. After transition, the actual birth of your baby will seem much easier.

Stage 2: Birth

PUSHING OUT YOUR BABY

Finally, you can push! You're completely dilated to 10 centimeters, and now is the time you'll be told that it's okay to push. After holding back in the earlier hours, it's a relief to many women to be able to actively push. Labor will feel less like something to bear now and more like something you can actively participate in. This is the labor we usually see on television shows—less managed pain, more pushing.

This stage of labor can last up to several hours for first-timers, but because you are actively engaged in *doing* something, you will be excited and probably get a big new surge of energy. If your contractions are strong enough, you will feel the baby bearing down on your rectum. Just as when you feel a big poop coming down, you will be unable to stop the overwhelming urge to get it out! Some women describe the opening of their body in this stage as a sexual feeling, but that wasn't my experience. For though it was intense, and extremely primal, it was painful. It was all about opening up as fully as possible to pass the baby out. I was sweating and had stripped naked. Wave after wave of pain washed over me, till I became the pain. I was squatting through most of my contractions, exhaling deeply as I did so, and I found myself closing my eyes, bobbing my head from side to side, and moaning occasionally. As I crouched, I clutched the railing of my brand-new changing table so hard I cracked it.

You hear a lot about screaming in birth horror stories, but I found that tuning into a silent place deep inside me kept me focused, and I was afraid that losing it by getting hysterical would send me in the wrong direction. Many women grunt, groan, sigh, or moan during labor, and you should make whatever sounds come naturally to you. If you find yourself more prone to screaming, try to take it down to a more guttural level. Screaming may just send you out of control, and it will waste your energy. Deep moaning works with your body's natural rhythms to help the baby emerge.

Contractions come very close together now, often without a break in between. Since you'll be working with the contractions now, they may not hurt as much as they did earlier. If your labor goes too slowly at this point, your doctor may want to speed things up with drugs like Pitocin. If you're at home, your midwives may give you herbs and pinch and rub your nipples. This pinching releases the natural hormone oxytocin, which encourages the uterus to contract. The baby's heartbeat will be monitored very closely now to check for any sign of distress. This is because, while labor is difficult for the woman laboring, it is also stressful for the baby making its journey out into the world. In particular, all the pushing and bearing down can be hard on the baby, and you may be given oxygen to supplement your own and the baby's supply. In the hospital, the baby's heartbeat may be measured by an electronic fetal monitor, but at home, a midwife can do it just as easily by using a stethoscope or Doppler. Although high-risk pregnancies require the use of a monitor, and they are handy for predicting contractions, they are unnecessary in most births.

THE BIRTH

You will now be in the room where you want to give birth, whether that's a birth pool, a hospital room, or your own bedroom. For me, attempting to lie on the bed (a standard hospital position) was an extremely painful thing. I simply could not do it, nor thankfully was I told I had to. I much preferred squatting down through the contractions while holding on to someone or something. When I felt the baby really coming, I moved over to the foot of my bed. With one foot perched on the low wooden footboard and one foot on the floor, I spontaneously went into what's called a "crescent moon" position, leaning over into a kind of squatting arch. Nothing could have moved me from this position once I assumed it. I found out afterward that this crescent moon shape is a position naturally assumed by women giving birth. My partner supported my weight in front, the midwives were ready to catch the baby, and everything seemed to be happening quickly, loudly, and intensely. Then the baby crowned.

When this happens, you will feel a burning sensation that some call "the ring of fire." I can see why. You feel absolutely stretched open, and it does hurt. At this point, many women in the hospital are given a cut through the perineum, called an *episiotomy,* to enlarge the opening, but most midwives advise against it. After all, women have been birthing babies forever, and there *is* enough room for a baby to pass through. Remember, don't let any doctor tell you this is a "routine" thing that all women need. You will not necessarily tear badly if you don't get an episiotomy. Even if you do tear, it may not be as bad as the deep cut you've been surgically given.

By the time you feel the head of your baby crown, or hear someone say "I can see the baby!" you're ecstatic to know you're almost done. After all you've been through, your baby is ready to be born! At this point, things happen super quickly. I remember midwife Deborah urging me, *"Push* your baby out, Rachel!" and then saying excitedly that she could see the head, and asking if I wanted to see it in a mirror. I said no, since I was seized with the incredible urge to just get that baby *out! Now!* And I kept pushing, while holding my partner in a vise grip, begging her not to move. Luckily, my mother took a picture at that exact second. It was a spellbinding moment, riding this huge wave of contractions, feeling the baby coming. It was everything you can imagine about the excitement of birth, all happening at lightning speed.

Then came the unbelievable, pure, blind sensation of a hard little head moving out of my vagina. She was just moving now on her own momentum into the world, and I could only ride it out. I felt her shoulders quickly push through, and as everyone was yelling "Here it comes!" the rest of her came tumbling out in a wet rush of goo. Then suddenly there was a baby lying face down next to me on the bed, struggling to breathe, making a tiny cry, attached to my body by a long curly purplish cord. My first, extremely eloquent, words upon seeing this wiggling, vernix-white-tinged but bloody little baby? "Oh my God, it's alive!" Brilliant, I know, and about all I was capable of after 24 hours of labor. And that's how Frances Ariel Pepper came into the world the night of August 19, 1998, drug-free, calm, and ready to suckle.

Of course, your baby's birth will be completely different from mine. Maybe you're having a C-section, or perhaps you're delivering multiples, or you've opted for pain medication, or you have complications that require a different kind of labor. If you're expecting a cesarean, or have health concerns that I haven't touched on, mainstream pregnancy books can provide the answers to other questions you might have. Whatever your experience, however, there will be that moment when you look at your baby for the first time and wonder at the miracle of birth. It sounds corny now, but it's true—you've managed to create this perfect tiny being, and the two of you are finally getting to meet. It's been a long time coming!

Stage 3: Afterbirth—Birthing the Placenta

DELIVERING THE PLACENTA

How anticlimactic! Yes, there is a third stage of labor. It is the passage of the placenta. By now, the cord has been cut, you've counted the baby's fingers and toes, and watched as he or she is cleaned up, weighed, and given an Apgar score. This test, administered a minute after birth and again at five minutes, measures the baby's color, heart rate, reflexes, muscle tone, and breathing. You've probably nursed the baby a bit, examined her hair color, and marveled at what a beautiful creature you've managed to create.

Probably the last thing you want to do at this point is push any more. The doctor or midwife may press your abdomen to see if the placenta is ready, and this may hurt. You may be dealing with small contractions and bleeding. To quell the bleeding you may be given an oxytocin shot. But the placenta must come out, so after a few pushes, it will separate from the uterine wall, and out will pop this rather grisly-looking but miraculous organ that fed your baby. Because I was very sore and had a tear, birthing the placenta was unpleasant, but I was nonetheless fascinated by how this deep-red and bloody "tree" had grown my newborn daughter.

The Incredible Placenta

All during your pregnancy, your blood has passed through the tissues of the placenta to give nourishment to the baby, and the baby's waste products and blood have passed back, to be processed by you. The placenta has also produced most of the hormones that ruled you the last nine months. Then, when it was time for the baby to be born, the placenta and uterus did a hormonal dance that, along with signals from the baby, triggers labor. Try not to be put off by the "ick" factor—take a look at this incredible organ. The side of it that was pressed against your uterus is rough, and the side that was turned toward the baby is smooth and cushiony. It looks like a giant piece of liver. It is the only organ your body can produce at will and then dispose of. Miraculous.

Various cultures honor the placenta in different ways. Here in North America, most placentas get tossed out with the rest of the hospital's organic waste, but you may wish to take yours home and bury it in some sort of ritual. Under a tree is a favorite place, I've heard. If I'd had a hospital birth, I probably would have left the placenta there, but my two midwives urged me to keep it. So I did, and it sat in the back of my freezer for a few years, awaiting a proper burial.

Some women also choose to bank their umbilical cord blood. This issue hardly existed when I had my daughter, but now it is big business.

A Midwife's Perspective on Hanky-panky During Labor
by midwife Deborah Simone, Awakenings Birth Services

A good part of the decision to birth at home with midwives involves choosing to avoid certain kinds of interventions. But there are also things to choose in favor of, such as privacy and familiarity. Birth is an extension of your sexuality. The greatest role your partner can play at your labor is one that she is already familiar with: that of your Lover. To labor in the circle of her love and support is the best kind of space for most laboring moms. This has nothing to do with timing contractions, ice chips, or rubbing your feet. It has everything to with the intimate space that belongs only to the two of you. The more relaxed, open, "juicy" a mom is, the better her labor will be. Oxytocin, the hormone that makes contractions, is the same hormone of arousal and orgasm. You are used to relaxing, responding, and opening to your lovers touch, what better labor tool? In my practice, we openly discuss incorporating sexual energy into the labor, something most of us would be unable to do in the hospital! Full body contact, massage that includes the breasts and vagina, masturbation and use of vibrators are all things to consider. Making sure that your midwives are comfortable with your expressions of sexuality is really important. Susie Bright once said that having a baby is like fisting in reverse! This means you can't rush the process, you gotta go nice and slow, and have lots of orgasms.

Cord blood may prove invaluable if your child, or even another family member, becomes very ill. You can arrange its storage in advance through a clinic or private company. If you are having a hospital birth, make sure your intention is known well in advance to everyone who will be in the room. Usually you need to buy a kit to collect the cord blood after the cord is cut. Even some sperm banks, like the California Cryobank, have accredited cord blood storage—their website includes a very concise explanation of this option. It costs upwards of $1200 to get your cord blood into a bank, and an additional, yearly fee for storage. For more general information on cord blood banking go to www.parentsguidecordblood.com.

Dealing with Complications

Of course, not every birth goes smoothly. Many women have complications of one kind or another somewhere along the way. This can include a "failure to progress" or even the need to induce labor, or problems involving the fetus. However, most complications can be dealt with fairly smoothly by both midwives and hospital staff, so don't let the thought of what *could* happen stress you out beforehand. Each birth takes its own course, and you *will* be able to cope with whatever comes up along the way. Even if you have a posterior-facing baby and end up with the dreaded and painful "back labor," or have a breech baby and perhaps need a cesarean, just remember that giving birth to your baby lasts only about a day, and after that you'll be able to enjoy the fruits of your labor for a lifetime.

> On the day we had our baby shower, five weeks before the baby was due, my partner said she didn't feel well. The next day we had a doctor's appointment, and once we got there our world went into a tailspin. They noticed a change in her blood pressure, and my partner's heart rate was accelerated. They put her on the fetal monitor and noticed that the baby's heart rate was dipping. Turns out the baby was breech, the amniotic fluid had disappeared, and the baby had not grown for a month. That is when the doctor looked at me and told me we'd need an emergency cesarean. They wheeled my partner into the emergency room and then cut away. I held her hand the entire time, while peeking over the screen to watch the operation. All of a sudden she

starts crying that we don't have a girl's name picked out yet, but at the same moment the doctor pulls out the baby's legs and says, "Don't worry about that, you have a boy!" —Erica

Partners Become Parents, Too

At the delivery you become a parent. One moment you're not and the next you are. The doctor will be finishing with your partner as you watch every move the baby makes while the nurses do their thing. You'll hover around the warming table and let the little hand wrap around your finger. It's an amazing transformation, just as profound for the person who didn't squeeze something that big out of a hole that small. How you got there is different, but once you're there it will matter very little to either of you.
—Sonia

In a few weeks after labor, you will have lost most of the vividness of the inseminations and the pregnancy. But the parent feeling will be there, and you'll never lose it! —Randye

For the partner of the pregnant woman, the birth of the baby is also a moving, life-changing event. Although she probably won't be called "Daddy" in the birthing room, what she will experience throughout labor and birth will be very similar to what men in heterosexual relationships go through. She may not be able to feel the contractions, but she will probably be there to help the laboring woman get through them. This kind of support is wonderful to have in labor, and if you have a partner, it's nice if she can be the one to give it to you. Make sure she knows you appreciate her, because she's working hard trying to make you more comfortable. In fact, although she can't feel your contractions, she'll be wincing every time you have one, worried both about your pain and how the baby is doing.

Partners should focus on keeping the birthing woman comfortable in any way she requests or requires. Breathe with her, massage her, and be as upbeat and supportive as possible. Especially as she hits transition, stay calm and encouraging, don't freak out, even if she does, and don't take anything she says or does now personally. If she has decided against pain medication, don't try to urge her to take any even if she's roaring like a lion. If she changes her mind and begs for some, don't stand in her way of it.

My midwife calls birth a transforming experience, and it certainly is for the partner, too. Any hesitations about sharing her life with a tiny baby usually disappear upon first glimpse of said child. Of course, the experience of getting through the birth may range from nerve-racking to deeply spiritual for the nonpregnant partner. It all depends on where the birth happens, whether there are any complications, and how soon everyone can be together afterward as a family. If the birthing woman is given a cesarean, the partner may well end up holding the baby first, during the stitching-up. Free from the overwhelming exhaustion and crashing hormones that a birthing woman experiences, the nonbiological mom can take full delight in the new baby. Any worries about bonding with the child generally fall away in a matter of hours.

The nonbiological mom should take over running the household while the birthing mom recovers, and she should feel welcome to hold the baby when it isn't nursing. Despite her good intentions, however, it's important that she never pressure the nursing mother by offering to bottle-feed the baby—to do "her share of the feeding." There are so many other useful chores the nonbio mom can do right now: change the baby, organize the household, do the cooking and laundry, phone anxious friends and family, take pictures and update the baby's website or your blog. All these things are part of running a family with a new baby in it. By being supportive in these ways, the nonbio partner allows the baby and mother to recover from the birth and develop a solid breastfeeding relationship— the most important gift you can currently give your newborn.

However, partners can also get overwhelmed. Too many chores and too little sleep? Maybe all you want to do as the supportive partner is watch your baby nurse, hold him when he sleeps, and be very close to your partner. So listen to what your heart tells you. Take some time off work, hire a housecleaner, and get friends to bring over some casseroles. This magic early time cannot be replaced. Be around for it.

A Few Pointers Still Ahead

Now that you've become parents, how do you take care of your incredible little creature? There are lots of books about newborn care, and I recommend a few in the resources section. You may feel stumped, but you probably know more than you think, as common sense and natural instinct go a long way in this parenting business. But turn the page for a few pointers, and then you'll be on your own very capable way!

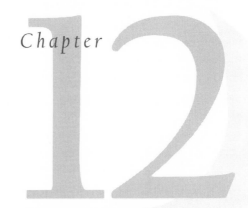

Chapter

Holy Cow—What Now?

Proud Passage to Lesbian Motherhood

The one thing on early mamahood I can say is, ask for people's help and sleep when the baby sleeps. That's what the midwife told us, and boy was she right! Sleep when the baby sleeps. —Nilda

What no one can fully realize beforehand is how a six-pound baby can come home with you from the hospital and completely take over your life. You won't feel like you have time to do anything— even go to the bathroom—those first few weeks. It's overwhelming. Joyful, but overwhelming. —Timotha

Well, you've done it! You're now well on your way to joining the proud ranks of lesbian mamas everywhere. Soon all this pregnancy and birth stuff will fade from memory, and you'll be wrapped up in the world of infants. Instead of obsessing with other women about ovulation kits and insemination timing, you'll be talking about how much weight your baby has gained, what kind of baby carrier you like, and how nursing is going.

Keep in mind that your baby's first weeks in this world are a rather surreal time for everyone in the household, particularly if this is your first child. This time is often called "the fourth trimester." The writer Sheila Kitzinger calls this lovely time "babymoon" and urges the birthing woman and her partner to stay restful, be loving, and learn about the baby. So put a sign on the door urging potential visitors to come back later: "Moms and baby are resting now." Keep things calm, focus on each other, and don't worry about the rest of the world.

There is a certain sense of astonishment that comes in the days after birth. This is when you realize that not only did your body create a brand-new human being, but this new person is here to stay—and you're solely responsible for it. Thank goodness for that initial rush of endorphins you have after birth—enjoy them while they last and get ready for what's to come. After about a week, things can get a little bit tougher.

Your newborn is so tiny, he or she seems so fragile, and you wonder how in the world you'll ever learn all you need to know about caring for this small but demanding creature. You're exhausted, and you're probably still a bit sore or bleeding from the birth. You're realizing how much there is to know about breastfeeding. You can't believe how night and day have taken on a strange new dimension, all a blur of diaper-changing, nursing, and napping. You might be fearful to go outside the house, because you feel so protective of the baby. Or you might be ready for your first walk outside, itching for things to feel back to normal, even while accepting that nothing will ever be back to the old normal again.

You're likely bursting with overwhelming emotion for the baby, and for your partner, if you have one. All this love, mixed with exhaustion and your sometimes confusing, conflicted feelings about the huge responsibility you now have, is almost more than you can take. Congratulations, you've joined the ranks of new moms everywhere!

What Is This Creature, Anyway? and Other Postbirth Revelations

As I wrote in the last chapter, the very first words out of my mouth, upon seeing my baby girl's dramatic exit from my flesh, were "Oh my God, it's alive!" Another woman I know said, "Shit, it's a baby!" You may laugh if you are reading this while still pregnant, but just you wait. Giving birth is strange enough, but seeing the creature you've nurtured inside of you for close to a year is a revelation. And usually it's a revelation not of profound love (that comes soon) but of astonishment. What *is* this tiny thing?

Newborns are rather ethereal creatures, and they remain so until they're about five or six weeks old. They're squirmy and almost opaque in color, they can't control their limbs or eyes, and they seem unbearably fragile and otherworldly. They make pathetically tiny, kittenlike cries and you can't imagine what they're asking for.

This creaturelike stage lasts only a few weeks. Soon you'll realize you don't exactly have a newborn any more, but an infant. The postpartum smoke will clear, you'll be back on your feet, and soon you'll get out of the house for short walks and errands. You'll start tromping around town with your baby in his carrier, and you'll realize that this baby feels a bit heavier, and looks quite a bit longer. Good goddess, are those really rolls of fat gathering on those previously scrawny legs? And could it be that this baby is actually looking right into your eyes, and smiling?

You'll realize that you've become more nonchalant and efficient about changing and burping your baby, and you're now a bit of a pro at nursing. Your nipples don't hurt anymore, and neither does your vagina. You know what all your baby's different cries mean, and you spend hours just gazing down at his or her sweet face, marveling at the hundreds of expressions that pass over it every minute.

Creature no more, your infant has become a sweet—but demanding—bundle of a baby. Your newborn has become a real little person already, and you've become a real mama. Congratulations, honey. I knew you could do it. And now the fun really begins.

New Mama Boot Camp

YOUR POSTPARTUM DO'S

- Nurse
- Sleep
- Watch talk shows
- Catch up on movies
- Read trashy magazines
- Eat healthy food
- Drink lots of water
- Take your vitamins
- Drink more water

- Have someone else cook and clean
- Bathe every day
- Change your clothes
- Change the baby's clothes

YOUR POSTPARTUM DON'TS
- Don't entertain too many guests
- Don't worry if the dishes pile up
- Don't give up on breastfeeding
- Don't watch violent TV shows or movies
- Don't worry about holding the baby "too much"
- Don't feel pressure to be perfect
- Don't feel pressured to have sex
- Don't feel pressured not to have sex if you want it and are able
- Don't freak out about how in the world you'll ever raise this tiny human being

Some Normal Early Considerations

Here are some things you might be concerned about in the first week or two. Some of these issues are painful, given that you wanted a child so badly. But all are normal, and all will pass quickly. I often tell parents that the first six months are new mama boot camp. There is so much to learn, and so many emotional touch-points to pass. Be gentle on yourselves, darlings, you'll get through it.

Can I Love This Baby?

It's weird to find out that after wanting to have a baby for years and trying so hard to create one, you might have some mixed feelings after its birth. Yet if you took a candid poll of a whole mix of different women, most would say they weren't passionately in love with their baby the moment it was born. Sure, they were feeling overwhelming emotions, and certainly much of it was love. But the all-encompassing mama-glow might not have come over you quite yet. For one thing, you've just had the most exhausting journey of your life, and you're too tired to feel much love for anyone. All you really want to do at the end of it is rest. Yet after what you've just been through, you're expected to bond immediately with this squirming little mess. Bonding takes time, and true love needs time to grow and deepen. You're not a bad person if you don't feel immediately like a loving mother. It's a new role, even if it's a much-awaited one. Allow yourself time to grow into the role of Mama, and soon you'll be madly in love with your little one. In fact, by the time she is eight weeks old and grinning at you with sheer adoration, you'll be wondering why you waited so long to have her, and when you can have your next one.

But What If It's a...?

No pregnancy book really likes to discuss the disappointment some women might feel about finding out at birth (or before, if you have genetic testing or ultrasounds) that the sex of the child they wanted is not the one they got. And the only writing on this subject from a lesbian perspective I'm aware of is Jess Wells's extremely honest and tender essay "Born on Foreign Soil," from her collection *Lesbians Raising Sons*.

Wells wanted a girl child so badly she paid to have the sperm she bought "sex-selected" to better the odds of having a girl. When a nurse pointed out the baby's penis during her amniocentesis, Wells was devastated. She writes, "I had been planning on a girl. It was essential that I have a girl...I was profoundly disappointed. I wept. I sobbed to my friends."

Now, surely, some readers may read this and say, "Ungrateful wench! I want a baby so badly I don't care what sex it is!" That's great, but some women do have a strong preference for one sex or the other. Indeed, many lesbians prefer to have a girl and just wonder what they'll do if they have a boy. In fact, it's almost an assumption among dykes that we prefer girl children, and we are always relieved when we have them.

Others, of course, long for a boy. I was in that smaller camp. I had always wanted boy children, assumed I would have boy children, and figured my odds of having one by donor insemination were pretty high. Since I had conceived right on the outer cusp of my ovulation, I knew, according to current thinking about insemination, that my odds of birthing a boy were good. My hopes were boosted by everyone who looked at me and swore that the way I was "carrying" meant I was having a boy. In particular I remember a very wise and beautiful woman who put her hands on my eight-months-pregnant belly and said, "I can tell you're having a boy. And I've never been wrong." In addition, I had bad morning sickness and pronounced hormonal mood swings, supposed signs of pregnancy with boys. Taking all this for confirmation, I told everyone it was a boy, agonized in excruciating detail over the choice of the perfect boy's name, and plotted the perfect future my boy and I would have together.

Was I surprised when the midwife turned the baby over and we saw that I had delivered a baby girl? You better believe it. I really wondered how this could have happened to me. My heart dropped in shock. How was this possible? Hadn't everyone said I was having a boy? Hadn't I wanted a boy child more than anything in the world? What was I going to do with a girl?

Well, there you have it. Hoping for one sex is a dangerous game: You may get the other. If you find out that your baby's sex is not the one you wanted, you will probably be disappointed for a few weeks, whether you find out at your baby's birth or during prenatal testing. It may help to remember that you wanted a child because you had so much love to give. And that love is still inside you, waiting for release.

It may also be a comfort to remember that, as lesbians, we don't have to box people, especially children, into rigid categories because of their sex at birth. There are many ways to be a girl and to be a boy. Similarly, there are many ways to raise one. Does it mean you can expect your girl—or boy—to love baseball as much as you and your partner do? That remains to be seen. Does it mean your boy—or girl— will love to shop and get his nails done? Maybe, maybe not. Personality is determined by genetics, environment, peer influence, and seemingly innate qualities that are unique to every individual. You are blessed to have the baby you have. As my midwife says, you get the baby you're meant to have, and surely yours is the perfect baby for you.

In hindsight, I know the grief I experienced over not birthing a boy child was real. As my daughter has grown up and I've grown as a mother, this grief has transmuted into an acknowledgment of all the wonderful things about having a daughter. At this point, my daughter and I are so bonded, and our lifestyle is so inherently female, that I cannot imagine now raising a boy. Flatteringly enough, my daughter is almost an exact minireplica of myself. She can even spot the one hot butch in a roomful of lesbians. What can I say? That's my girl.

Jess Wells, in the essay quoted above, remarks that a year after her amnio she found all her apprehensions about having a son "inconse-quential." She writes, "My son is here. I am so in love with him and so bound to him that I would do anything to make his life joyous, healthy and safe." Whether you hope to have a boy, a girl, or simply don't care, no doubt you will feel the very same way.

The Intersex Possibility

There is yet another possibility to consider. I have never seen this mentioned in any other pregnancy or parenting book, but it is a fact: Some children are born intersex. *Intersex* is an umbrella term for a whole range of people born with genitals that are not considered exactly male or female. A baby boy could be born with what is called a "micropenis," or a girl with an unusually large clitoris, or the child could be born with some combination of what we think of as male and female genitalia. According to the statistic that is often cited, one in every 2,000 births is an intersex birth.

In the past, this topic was shrouded in secrecy and shame. Parents who were faced with this surprising reality at the birth of a newborn had no advance information about it and didn't know how to respond. Usually they were put under extreme pressure by doctors to "choose" a sex for their infant, often the one the doctor recommended, and that was usually female. This was considered "normalizing" the child through surgery, though such children often grow up feeling a mismatch between their sex and their gender identity.

Today, in response to groups like ISNA—the Intersex Society of North America (online at www.isna.org)—the medical establishment has shown more understanding of intersex people. If you, as a new parent, have an intersex newborn and face decisions such as this, seek guidance from others who have gone before you. Consult the ISNA website, or Bodies Like Ours (www.bodieslikeours.org), which has specific information for new parents and can help you find people to talk to about this. You have no obligation to act immediately to provide surgery that will "fix" your child; resist any pressure to do so. As I learn more about intersex people, I more fully appreciate the enormous continuum of human sexuality, and the potential for differences among us.

Getting Help

There will be many times, especially when your infant is crying inconsolably, when you feel like tearing your hair out. A lot of newborns cry a lot, and this can be frustrating. It's hard enough when there are two or more grown-ups in the house. A partnered lesbian whose spouse is at work will feel quite helpless at these times, and single mothers may really grapple with isolation. It's easy to see how new mothers become over-whelmed—inexperience, isolation, and lack of sleep combined with the constant demands of a newborn can just be too much. When things get bad, the best thing a mom can do is pick up the phone and call a friend, or reach out to other moms online. (A childless friend will try to be sympathetic, but won't really get it. I recommend trying to reach another mom.)

The other lifesaver is to simply change the scene. Put the baby in a front pack and go for a walk. Or load him up in the car and get to a play-ground. Have a cup of tea in a café, with other real, live grown-ups. Briefly visit a nearby museum or store. Linger in places where you might find other new moms. They'll fawn over your newborn, and you'll feel a big sense of relief and the warmth of a community. Knowing when you're reaching your limit—and we all have one—will help keep both you and your newborn happy.

Postpartum Problems

It's normal to experience crashing hormones after the birth of a baby. The first few days, you'll float in a cloud of euphoria, amazed that your labor has produced a real, live human being. You'll tell everyone you're just fine, you'll feel energetic, entertain guests, and then…you'll crash. Exhaustion, lack of sleep, a crying baby, no milk, and a sore body can contribute to this. It is sometimes called "the baby blues," or "third day comedown." Most women cry, long for sleep, and can't believe their discomfort. Who told them this is what it was like to be a mother? Take comfort, my friends, this period normally doesn't last long.

However, if you find that your crashing postbirth hormones, lack of sleep, physical discomfort, and the demands of a newborn are all too much, and this feeling lasts more than a few weeks, pay attention. This could be postpartum depression. I'd say it's pretty common to experience a touch of it. Luckily, this topic has gone from taboo to talk show. Now even celebrity moms like Brooke Shields talk about it.

Women who have hospital births tend to be more susceptible to postpartum depression than women who've had home births. After you give birth at home, you have a midwife who comes and checks on you almost every day. But when you give birth in the hospital, once you're sent home you're usually on your own. Support for a new mother is so important, and it is not given the respect it deserves in our culture. Women are just expected to know how to cope with a newborn, often while alone and isolated, for many hours at a time. In other countries, where a new mother is surrounded by female relatives and friends, postpartum depression is not so much an issue.

If you find that you have lingering feelings of depression after the birth of a baby, you might need help. Some anxiety is normal with a newborn in the house, but you may experience panic attacks, an uncontrollable fear of the baby dying, or even urges to hurt the baby or yourself. All these feelings require professional help. But it is helpful to remember that a hormonal or biochemical imbalance is often the cause of postpartum depression. There are first-person accounts of postpartum depression online and numerous books about the topic, including Brooke Shields's honest and moving *Down Came the Rain*. If you think you might fit the profile for postpartum depression, don't be ashamed to reach out for help. Groups like the La Leche League, an advocacy group that promotes breastfeeding, can be a good place to start. Hiring a doula in the early postnatal weeks can help alleviate your isolation and feelings of frustration.

How a Doula Can Help

I like to describe the role of a doula as a professional equivalent to how women used to care for each other during the nineteenth century. Mothers, aunts, and neighbor ladies all supported the mother in birth and then helped her afterward to keep the home running. Now we hire doulas to fill that role. It can be a real lifesaver for a new mom. —Arlene

Consider hiring a doula to take care of you and your baby for the first week or two. I have stressed this in previous chapters, and for good reason. Doulas are trained to care for new mothers and their babies. They don't come to your home to ooh and ahh over the baby, nor do they expect you to entertain them. They are there for you. Besides cooking and cleaning for you and making sure you're comfortable, they can answer questions about breastfeeding and ensure that you're healing properly. They also provide precious reassurance to a new mom that she's doing a good job and will soon be on her feet. This kind of caregiving, so important to new moms, has typically been the domain of female relatives. But many women today, without an extended network of support around them, consider a doula the best two-week investment they ever made for themselves. The services of a doula can significantly lower the risk of isolation and postpartum depression.

The Milk Bar's Always Open

Breastfeeding has been an amazing experience for me. Sitting with my daughter, seeing little drops of milk at the corner of her mouth as she suckles, still gives me butterflies in my stomach. —Riley

Prior to my daughter's birth, I would never give myself quiet time to just sit, relax, and reflect. During our feeding sessions, there's little else to do but watch the beauty and perfection of my daughter. I enjoy this time together as much as she does! —Fatima

Breastfeeding Is the Best Choice

Both for you and for your baby, breastfeeding is the best choice you can make. It is best for you because it helps you bond with your baby, helps your body heal faster, and it's cheap, always available, and a whole lot less fuss than formula. I think, too, that it's one of the most amazing aspects of being a new mother, this incredible ability to make the perfect food for your child.

The main reason to breastfeed, of course, is that it's best for your baby. Breast milk is, quite simply and without argument, the perfect first food. Your body instinctively knows just the right kind of milk to produce for your particular baby. The composition of your milk changes depending on your baby's age, and even over the course of a single feeding. The first milk a mother releases is sweet, to entice the baby to stay latched on. Later in the feeding, she produces the rich hind milk, which is higher in nutrients and also helps a baby poop. Breast milk contains natural antibodies that strengthen your baby's immune system, help prevent future allergies in your child, and may actually make your baby smarter than formula-fed babies. Breastfed babies get fewer ear infections, and fewer gastric problems, and they are also less likely to become lactose intolerant later on.

In short, breastfeeding is just about perfect.

Of course, there are women to whom breastfeeding may seem undesirable. Perhaps the thought of a baby latched on to your breast seems strange, or inconvenient. Or perhaps you and your partner have decided that bottle-feeding will make things more "equal" between you. It's true, too, that some women have terrible difficulty breastfeeding, or can't seem to produce enough milk.

If you choose not to breastfeed, or find you just can't do it, you're not a bad person, or a terrible mother. Formula will nourish your baby, and bottle-feeding a baby can also be a highly intimate experience.

However, bottle-feeding comes in a distant second to the miracle of breastfeeding. Like many worthwhile things in life, breastfeeding is work at first. It takes patience, practice, and a certain amount of self-sacrifice and initial discomfort. It's a skill that both you and your baby have to learn—together. There are entire books devoted to the topic of breast-feeding. I urge you to have, in particular, *The Nursing Mother's Companion* by Kathleen Huggins on hand—it explains all aspects of breastfeeding in scrupulous detail. And if you have any questions about nursing, the La Leche League is there to help you, and they're only a phone call away (1–800-LA-LECHE, or visit their web-site at www.laleche.org).

Breast-feeding may be "natural" but it is also a skill that both you and your baby must learn. The early weeks can be hard, but it will get easier with time and effort.

Techniques and Tips for Nursing

Here is the best advice I can give you in the early stages of breastfeeding: Make sure that both you and your baby are correctly positioned. You should be sitting up comfortably in bed or in a chair with adequate back support. Use a specialty cushion or pillow to help you hold the baby high enough. Hold him close to your body in a position that cradles him right in front of you. Then guide his mouth toward your breast—without moving forward or slouching. If he resists, brush your nipple against his mouth. (Tandem feeding with twins works a bit differently, with a child held on each side of you.) There are photos of nursing mothers in many breast-feeding books and websites, so use them for inspiration.

Proper positioning helps with the "let-down" release that lets the milk flow. If you are not in the right position, the baby can suckle just your nipple, rather than draw your breast all the way in toward the back of his mouth. This extension of your nipple is what makes nursing work. And this is why your nipple and areola—no matter how big or small, should seem to disappear entirely into the baby's mouth as he suckles. Your nipple is actually drawn down to the middle of his palate. His lips should be parted, and his nose will be pressed down almost flat against your breast. A small newborn baby will look almost squashed against you. Don't worry, breastfeeding won't suffocate the baby!

Set up a nursing station in a comfortable, upright chair, with a basket of necessary items at your side. These include a book or magazine, a bottle of water and some snacks, nipple cream, and a cordless phone. This way, you won't be "stuck" during a long feeding session, unable to get a drink or answer an important call.

If your positioning is wrong, and you need a quick way to get the baby to let go of your nipple, don't just pull him off. Instead, slide a clean finger into the side of the baby's mouth—he should let go enough for you to separate. Then try repositioning yourself. This technique can also be used to detach a baby who has fallen asleep at the breast but is still latched on. Remember to alternate your breasts, either during a feeding or from one feeding to the next. Sometimes babies favor one side. Do what you can to discourage this in early nursing by offering the less-favored breast first.

Here Comes the Milk

During her first few days of life, when your baby nurses she will only get small amounts of a premilk substance called colostrum. It's a thick, gel-like liquid rich in protein and infection-fighting properties. Colostrum also helps the baby, while it is still a fetus, pass its first meconium poop, and it primes baby's intestines with healthy flora to aid in digestion. It's only produced by the body for a short time, and it's a miracle substance no formula can ever copy. Keep putting the baby to your breast, even if your milk hasn't come in yet. This will help the milk come, usually around the third to the fifth day postbirth.

The arrival of your milk is a cause for celebration. What no one told me, though, was that sometimes accompanying this event is a terrible, albeit temporary, condition called engorgement. Engorgement hurts. I didn't cry once during my whole labor, but I wept when my breasts got engorged. It can feel like two huge, hard melons are sitting on your chest where your breasts used to be. This happens because, not only are your breasts stuffed with milk, your body's sense of supply and demand is still out of whack. Once you become engorged, the only way to prevent losing your milk supply or getting an infection of the breast called mastitis is to get the milk out.

Unfortunately, your breasts may be so full that you can't even latch the baby on to suckle. Many women use a breast pump for this problem, but I found a solution that worked just as well: having my lover suck at my breasts to drain them. This was definitely one of the more hilarious moments of my childbirth experience, though at the time it was an act of desperation. If you and your partner are willing to try this, it is easier and cheaper than renting a pump. You can also try applying warm or cold compresses (such as a package of frozen peas). I found standing under a hot shower also really helped my milk start to flow.

Some babies instinctually root around, heads bobbing, mouths wide open, as soon as they're put near warm flesh. They're like a cute baby bird, pecking around, waiting to be fed. One of my daughter's early nick-names was actually "Birdie" for this reason. Other babies take a little longer to get the hang of breastfeeding. To help such a baby, stroke her cheek to get her to turn her head toward you. Then touch her lip or chin to get her to open up that little mouth. As soon as she does, jam the baby's head right onto your breast, making sure she has as much of your nipple and areola in her mouth as possible. Remember, if the baby takes just the nipple, she's not really getting any milk. Worse yet, you will end up in incredible pain, and your hungry baby will be frustrated and probably crying hysterically. After a few days you'll be able to tell in a few seconds if she's latched on properly.

Don't forget to burp your baby after every feeding. A few gentle pats on the back while he is pressed against your shoulder usually does the trick. You'll figure out quickly the best way of burping your baby. It's important to burp until you hear a nice big belch, so gas doesn't build up in that tiny digestive system and cause discomfort.

How much milk is enough to feed your baby? If your baby is gaining weight, eating eight or ten times a day, regularly wetting at least six diapers a day, and is content after a feeding, your baby is most likely getting enough to eat.

Don't Schedule Feeding; Feed on Demand

It's very important that you not try to put your baby on any feeding schedule. Rather, feed on demand. Some people believe you can "train" a baby when to eat, just as you can "train" it to sleep. Both of these beliefs are mistaken. Babies are not capable of rational thought. A newborn's driving force is simple survival. For this it needs the gentle touch of its mother and constant access to breast milk. A baby has a tiny tummy and must eat frequently in order to survive and thrive. Most newborns feed at least eight times a day, for up to 45 minutes at a time.

It May Hurt in the Beginning, but Don't Give Up

Most books tell you that breastfeeding doesn't, or shouldn't, hurt. This is unfortunately not true for certain stages of the breastfeeding experience. The pain may be bad in the beginning, as you learn how to nurse. You also may experience very normal uterine cramping from nursing during the first week. As your nipples toughen up from this new experience, it should cease to hurt. This can take several weeks, or even several months. The discomfort can be made worse by conditions such as thrush, by cracked or bleeding nipples, and by improper positioning. During this sensitive time, make sure you wear a soft nursing bra or no bra, don't use soap to wash your breasts, and know there are special creams you can buy to relieve your poor, sore nips. Pure lanolin is a good salve.

I remember, in my early breastfeeding experience, I found the going very tough. There was a period during the first few weeks when my right nipple was very sore, and I can remember wincing from the pain. When Frances nursed during that time, it felt like a dagger slicing me inside from my nipple to my shoulder. Similarly, my friend Emily recalls lying awake in the night nursing her son, tears running down her face from the pain. Other women can't believe how their breasts leak milk all over the place, even just from hearing someone else's baby cry.

All these factors can make women give up on breastfeeding before they ever get the hang of it. But if you can make the commitment to stick it out for about six weeks, you'll become an old pro very quickly. Remember when I said breastfeeding was a learned skill? Besides learning how to position your baby and get in tune with its needs, your nipples also have to learn to toughen up. Once they do, in a few short weeks, nursing becomes a very pleasant experience, deeply satisfying on both a physical and emotional level. You'll find, as you get more experienced and your baby gets a bit bigger, that you're able to nurse in a variety of other positions as well. This can include a football hold, sideways lying down, and even half-asleep while you and your baby cuddle up in bed.

You can probably tell by now that there's a lot to learn about breastfeeding. Yes, it may be a natural function, but it's not a skill that comes "naturally" to all first-time mothers. Don't be discouraged if it's a bit harder than you initially thought. I just can't emphasize enough that it is well worth the effort. There's nothing like relaxing on a cozy couch and gazing down at the satisfied face of your baby suckling at your breast. It's a proud moment when you realize you have cleared the early hurdles and have become a pro at this.

Nursing Gear and Attitude

As far as breastfeeding, accessibility, and fashion go, these are all a matter of your personal comfort level. Some women are embarrassed to nurse in public. Ladies, never let anyone make you feel that by feeding your baby you are doing something wrong. Community standards on this subject vary depending on where you live, but it's up to us to push the envelope. Essentially, you should be able to nurse wherever and whenever you need to; laws in many states dictate that a nursing mother cannot be asked to move. I was timid at first, but by the time Frances was a few months old I was proudly nursing wherever I wanted. This included standing behind the counter at my small store, holding my nursing baby with one hand and ringing up customers' sales with the other! I'll never forget the look on some (usually male) customers' faces when this occurred, but I didn't care. It was my business, and this was my baby, and I was going to nurse. Chalk one up for the cause of nursing moms' visibility!

When you are out and about with a new baby, it can be hard not to take comments about your nursing personally. One of the most common is "Can't you do that in the bathroom?" It helps to have a comeback line ready, such as "Would YOU want to eat your lunch in the bathroom?" Until the U.S. catches up with other countries and provides dedicated, clean, and comfortable areas for nursing moms to feed their babies, you will have to do what you can.

You can certainly wear everyday clothes while breastfeeding, but happily, there are companies that make specially designed nursing clothes. One of the largest is Motherwear, at www.motherwear.com. They sell mostly T-shirts and dresses, all with variously designed slits or flaps that you pull open and pop your nipple and a small portion of your breast through. It's wise to invest in at least one or two of these, as well as a supportive nursing bra. These are different from everyday bras, extremely comfortable and absorbent for leakage. Many maternity stores now have nursing bras, but one of my favorites is Bravado Designs, started by two young moms to provide good quality and more funky styles to nursing moms. Their website is www.bravadodesigns.com. Some places also sell special tentlike cloths to drape over the baby, so you can hide your booby while you nurse. I find these attract more attention than simply sitting there nursing.

Always have some burp cloths around when you nurse, since spit-up is a fluid you'll become very familiar with. It's also good to have a diaper ready if you're going to breastfeed—nursing often triggers a baby to poop.

For nursing advice, ask your doctor or midwife, or call the La Leche League (1–800-LA-LECHE) or visit their website at www.laleche.org. They can also locate a volunteer in your area to come over and help you in the beginning stages. I took advantage of this wonderful service and recommend it to you, so don't be shy.

Alternating bottle-feeding with nursing can cause your baby nipple confusion. This is because it requires a completely different technique for a baby to drink from a piece of hard rubber than from a pliant human nipple. The milk flows differently as well—breastfeeding takes more effort on the baby's part. He or she will likely become frustrated by the difference and end up refusing the breast. To avert an abrupt and deeply disappointing weaning, do not bottle-feed at all for the first few months.

If You Bottle-Feed

Bottle-feeding is a second-best alternative to breastfeeding, but it is one some women prefer. It can also be an intimate experience for moms and babies. Make sure you mix the formula well, and don't heat the bottle in the microwave—it could heat unevenly and burn the baby's mouth. Hold your baby close and make it a restful, nourishing time for both of you. Never leave the baby alone with a bottle propped up in his mouth— he could choke.

For the Partner

If you're the partner of the birth mother, you're probably exhausted too. You're also feeling incredibly excited and maybe even scared about what this new little person will mean to your life. Make sure you are able to get your rest, especially if you're the one working outside the home every day to pay the bills. Don't expect to be able to work full time and then come home and take care of your partner and the baby every night, and do amazingly large loads of laundry, and not be exhausted. If you are able to find willing helpers, line up friends and family, or hire someone else to cook and clean so you can enjoy your time with your partner and newborn. Instead of racing around doing the shopping, give your wife a foot rub, read her a story, or take care of the baby so she can have a nap. Since it's almost impossible for a new mom to separate herself from a newborn for more than a few minutes, she will be counting on you to hold the baby so she can take a much-longed-for shower or bath.

Whatever you do, don't pressure the nursing mother in any way or interfere with the breastfeeding experience. Being supportive also includes not making light of the hard work it takes to breastfeed a child. It can be exhausting and physically unnerving in the beginning as baby and nursing mom figure it all out. For many first-time mothers, breast-feeding an infant is a whole-body experience. It's not like turning on a tap. Sensitivity and support in dealing with a new mom as she learns to nurse will do much to earn a breastfeeding mom's gratitude.

Your role during this time is to encourage and respect the intimate ritual that nursing becomes for the biological mother and child. Help your partner get comfortable, bring her a glass of water or juice, and help keep the mood mellow. She'll be hungry, since breastfeeding requires additional calories. So bring her some healthy snacks, and don't make cracks about her gaining more weight. You can take the baby after he nurses and burp him, and hold him while he sleeps. In a few short months, your partner can express some milk, and you can try bottle-feeding. Before you know it, your baby will be six months old, eating solid foods, and the feeding dynamic will have changed dramatically. Don't try to rush this process because of your own impatience. Introducing a bottle too early may lead to nipple confusion for the baby and mean an end to breastfeeding.

Partners should also keep in mind that birthing women are potential time bombs of crashing hormones. This may mean she'll go a little nutty for a few weeks as her body adapts and she adjusts to the demands of an infant. Be as loving as you can, and know that your partner appreciates everything you do for her, even if she can't express it right now. And remember, by being kind to your partner and taking care of her right now, you are also doing what's best for the baby.

Your Body—the Birth Battleground

No one really tells you that getting a C-section is having major surgery. It's not like spraining your ankle. It was painful for weeks afterward. I'd rather go through a weeklong labor next time than have another cesarean. —Lisa

I assumed I'd be back at work in a matter of days after the birth. Surprise! I would never have believed that I could bleed for weeks afterward. I had to learn that it takes time to heal. —Carlin

Some people may take offense at the analogy of your body as a battleground. But once you've had a child, you'll probably be able to relate to it. Whether you've had a C-section and are recovering from this major surgery or have had a vaginal birth, your body will never be quite the same. Your vagina is ripped and sore and the size of a football. There's blood everywhere, your tits are about to burst, your skin's flapping around on your tummy, and you're wondering if you'll ever be able to poop again. Sure, childbirth may be a "natural" event, but you won't feel so natural afterward for a few weeks.

When you are postpartum, there's nothing you can really do about all this. Allowing yourself to rest and recover is the only remedy for basic childbirth trauma. Requiring you to stay in bed for a week or two, or even more, may be nature's way of making sure you stay close to your baby. If all you had to do was pop it out and continue on your way, the human species could not have survived.

Sure, there may be women among us who can have a baby and run a marathon the next week. They're probably 20 years old and in great shape. For the rest of us, healing will take longer. The amount of time depends on your age, physical condition, and what kind of birth you had. Listen to your doctor's or midwife's advice about the best path to healing for you. Remember to use a squirt bottle of water to gently clean your vaginal area after using the toilet. Take sitz baths to soothe your sore self and calm any hemorrhoids. Herbal remedies, and homeopathic ones such as arnica, are a new-mother's salve. Learn about them and use them. New mothers can be very susceptible to infection from their birth wounds or cesarean scars. Use antiseptic procedures as much as possible without becoming obsessive about it. Drink lots of water to ease constipation, and use chilled sanitary pads (keep some in the freezer) to soothe a swollen perineum. Don't jerk your body around too quickly in bed, and don't try to do laundry five days postpartum, as I did. You will regret it, as I did, if you break open a tear that is healing.

Your vagina may feel and look very freakish after your baby's natural birth. The swelling will go down soon, and things will get back almost to normal within a few months. Sure, you may have a new skin flap, or some scarring, but this is part of having a kid, along with possible stretch marks, bigger hips, and a squishier tummy. Consider yourself indoctrinated into the mama body hall of fame. Your body is especially sacred now—it created human life.

Will I Ever Sleep Again?

You won't sleep very much in the early postpartum period. The first two weeks will be a time of difficult adjustment for the baby, and therefore for you. Accustomed to short cycles of activity and rest inside the womb, the baby will take some time getting used to the rhythms of the outside world. Count on the baby sleeping in two-to-three-hour segments during the early weeks, with several feedings throughout the night. This is why we tell new moms, "Sleep when the baby sleeps." It may be the only sleep you get.

Don't be fooled by some people's accounts of having "easy" babies who sleep through the night right from the start. This is so rare it's laughable. It also doesn't take into account the difference between bottle-fed babies (who sometimes sleep more easily through the night) and breastfed babies, who need to feed much more frequently. Be aware, too, that an "easy" baby can change dramatically as it enters the next stage of development, and that a baby's sleep rhythms also change from month to month.

Yes, sleep deprivation can wipe you out. In particular, you won't get enough deep sleep, and this can take its toll. Keep in mind that extreme sleep deprivation is a time-limited phenomenon. It will peak at several months and slowly ease up till the baby's about a year old. At one year, most babies can sleep through the night. If you have a partner, try to tag-team your sleep in the beginning so you're not both exhausted all the time.

On Attachment Parenting

Our son used to cry so much as a baby, we started bringing him into bed with us. He just seems to sleep better that way. And that means we are sleeping better too! —Libby

Take a hint from native cultures that keep their babies with them all the time. We are mothers and its our job to mother. Please don't think about having a child and then shoving it into a room by itself for the next eighteen years. Keep your babies close and they'll grow up, as mine has, to be happy, independent children with lots of self-esteem. —Alma

Get some sort of pouch to carry your baby with you on your body. They love it and you'll be more connected than if you just plop your baby in a stroller. —Heidi

The idea of attachment parenting has been gaining popularity in North America in recent years. The funny thing is, a practice we are only now studying and giving a name to is simply how most of the world raises its children. Attachment parenting really just promotes the idea of spending lots of time together with your baby—being literally attached to her as well as finely tuned in to her—as you provide for your baby's innate needs. This includes breastfeeding, sleeping with your baby, carrying him on your body in a carrier or sling, and doing things a bit more low-tech than modern parents generally do. Many lesbians lean towards this style of parenting, to varying degrees.

I found that attachment parenting was a natural fit for me. I loved carrying baby Frances in her sling, being with her almost every moment, and breastfeeding on demand. I never questioned my instinct to hold my baby, pick her up when she cried, or keep her close to me at night. Attachment parenting is a philosophy of the heart, and it teaches you to go with your instincts. For example, you know as a parent that if your child cries, you'll want to reach for her and pick her up. This response is imprinted in our genetic code; as a species we would not have survived without it. When people give you bad advice, such as telling you not to "spoil" your baby or nurse him "too much," ignore them. Childless people don't know what they're talking about, and older relatives may have outdated ideas about childrearing. Babies need all the love and attention we can give them. This helps them grow up as secure and happy people who are capable of loving others. There will be lots of time later for order, discipline, and schedules.

Cosleeping with the Peppers

Cosleeping, a term that really just means sleeping with your baby in a family bed, is probably the biggest topic of controversy in parenting circles. Here are some myths about cosleeping, dispelled. First, some people think you'll suffocate the baby if you sleep with it. This is not true. Unless you're taking sleeping medication or engaging in drugs or heavy drinking, there is little risk of rolling over onto the baby. In fact, most babies are safer sleeping next to you—the risk of SIDS (sudden infant death syndrome) is much lower in babies who cosleep. I believe the reason for this is that a baby in the same bed can feel, smell, and hear its parents, and its breathing may be more regular as a result. Second, some people feel cosleeping is not a socially acceptable behavior. In fact, in most of the world, parents sleep with their young children. It makes it easier for mothers to breastfeed and can be a lovely bonding time for parents who are separated from their babies during the day.

My own story of cosleeping with my daughter is a fairly typical one. As a newborn, baby Frances was very close by—often sleeping right on my tummy. By a week or two old, she slept draped over me, her head often on my breast, ready to nurse. At a few months old, when she was getting heavier, she could be found curled up by my side, a warm and sweet-smelling little bundle. When she entered a kicking phase and I was desperate for sleep, she would go in her cradle.

Around four months old, she graduated to a crib in my bedroom, but would often join me in the night for nursing and sleep there till morning. On and off through her toddler years, she would be in and out of my bed. If anyone needed more space it was usually me, depending on whether I had a girlfriend or simply needed some solo sleeping time. When I bought my house, she finally got her own bedroom, and I was ready for a bit more solid, childfree sleep.

Now in elementary school, my daughter is firmly ensconced in her own bedroom, with her big-girl twin bed, complete with a fluffy Hello Kitty blanket and all manner of pink pillows. Often, she still taps on my door in the middle of the night, hoping for an invitation in. Sometimes, I call out to her to go back to her own bed, and she will do so with no fuss. Other times, if I open the door, she'll be standing there, beloved blankie in hand, ready to run across the room and hop into "Momma's bed." Sometimes I let her sleep with me, but it never becomes a habit. In winter, I admit, she's as comforting and warm as a hot-water bottle.

This push and pull of cosleeping has evolved organically for us. There have been some rough patches and backsliding, but all in all, I feel I have done well by both of us. I have no regrets about our cosleeping career, or the gentle way we have gradually weaned ourselves apart. My child sleeps well through the night now, and so do I. There are few nightmares in our house.

Because I am a single mom, this experience has been different from how a couple would work things out. Couples will rightly feel that they need a little more private time at night without the baby. Differences may arise, with one partner more resistant to a "no baby in the bed" policy, but usually a solution can be worked out. Perhaps the nursing mom will fall asleep with the baby, and then the baby will be moved to a different room, or a nearby crib. Be flexible, and try to keep a sense of humor about it. Most important, listen to your heart, and try to get some sleep!

The Beauty—and the Difficulty—of Becoming a Family

One of the sweetest times in my life was the period immediately after Noah was born. It was then that my partner and I realized that for better or for worse, we were now a family. All of the

expense and work of trying to get pregnant and the whole difficult pregnancy was behind me. I had actually given birth to a baby! My endorphins buzzed, my hormones still flew high, and I was damn proud of the way I had labored and delivered my baby.
—Judy

We broke up a month after Ryan's birth. It was just too hard on our relationship. Now I'm a single mom, and she sees him on Saturdays. —Val

Whatever kind of birth you have, try to enjoy the postdelivery period. Soon you'll be dealing with a parade of visitors, your body will be a wreck, and you won't sleep for weeks. You may also find that your relationship with your partner goes through some hard times now. The initial euphoria of birth may give way to a time of tension as you work out your roles as new parents. Whether you're coparenting with your partner, whether she's the dyke daddy and you're the acknowledged mom, or even whether there are more than two of you as parents, there will probably be a shakedown. It will take some time to figure things out. It can be easier for a single mother in this respect, since she does not have to negotiate with a partner about various duties and roles. It takes time to grow as a family, whatever your orientation, and no matter how many people are involved. But, being queer, we have the freedom to create new kinds of family structures and not be constrained by the more rigid boundaries of the straight world.

Only you—and your partner, if you have one—can decide what kind of family you want to create. Remember that a family can be created in many ways, and that all families grow and change with time.

If you're in a coupled relationship, it's particularly important to keep the lines of communication open. Don't stop talking about the changes you and your relationship are going through. Expect a period of adjustment, and trust that you'll be able to navigate through all of this. Do keep in mind, however, that having a baby is a bit like throwing a bomb into the middle of your life. You can't just pick up and carry on as things were before. Some couples, particularly in newer relationships, don't survive such an explosion.

But, for now, just enjoy the tremendous gift of your new baby, and don't worry too much about tomorrow.

Basic Baby Care—Learning with Love

Fortunately, your little one won't care how much or how little you know; they only need to know that you're there for them. My first words to my daughter, after "I'm so glad you're here," were "Well, I guess we'll figure this out together." And we did. —Robin

You're almost ready to head out into the wonderful world of lesbian mothering. Soon, instead of reading pregnancy books, you'll be perusing baby and child-care books. You will barely give a thought to those pre-conception or pregnancy days, unless you decide to go through all this again. And if you do, you'll have a lot of valuable experience under your belt that will make it much easier the second, or third time, through.

The needs of your newborn are really quite simple: to sleep, to be kept warm and comfy, and to be fed, changed, and held as much as possible, all with love and interaction. You will have to learn your own baby's cues and how to respond to them, which will seem daunting in the first few weeks. But let me reassure you that much of being a good mama is instinctual, and the more you go with the flow, the easier things will get. Don't be afraid of your baby. If your newborn is full term, she has already made it through nine months of life and is ready to be with you. So take in some "expert" advice, mix it with what your heart and gut tell you, and most of all, *enjoy* being a mother.

Where to Go from Here, in Short

Get a diaper bag, pack it, put the baby in his sling or carrier, and start heading back out into the world. Go slowly at first. Join a new-mom support group, or start one—this may quickly become a highlight of your week. Go for walks. Take a mommy and baby yoga class. Read nonfiction antholo-gies about life as a new mom. Slowly integrate yourself into the world of motherhood and its myriad activities. Your life will be different now: You are a mother. You are up to the challenge. Be gentle with yourself. Look to empathetic child-care books and trusted mom friends for advice.

A Parting New-Mama Message from Aimee Gelnaw
Executive Director, Family Pride Coalition, 2001–2005

Welcome to one of the most loving, committed, and intentional parenting communities. Fortunately for you, the LGBT parenting community is growing and flourishing and offers myriad opportunities to learn, celebrate in community, and advocate for a just and welcoming world for our families and children. The Family Pride Coalition is the national not-for-profit organization whose mission is to promote equality for LGBT parents and their families. As a national community we have much work to do and know that we succeed only when we do this together. Family Pride supports local parenting groups nationwide and offers resources for families on issues most relevant to parenting such as talking to children about our families, making schools safe for our kids, considering and planning your family, building a local parenting group, and many others. The website (www.familypride.org) provides information and resources related to advocacy, education, and support and offers opportunities to get involved in both social and advocacy related opportunities. Annual events such as Family Week in Provincetown, Massachusetts, provide opportunities to network, find support, learn, and work together. An e-newsletter keeps our national community connected and informs members of ways to be involved such as addressing unjust legislation, finding community resources, and keeping abreast of the issues relevant to our family movement. Family Pride sponsors a research symposium in conjunction with a major university illuminating research on our families and providing those who serve our families with the information needed to ensure our well-being in our towns, communities of faith, schools, legislatures, and in all of the arenas that impact our selves and our children. Once again, welcome, and congratulations on your courageous and loving decision to bring children into the world.

My Final Congrats

You've certainly come a along way since the early chapters of this book, when your biggest concern was checking your fertile mucus. Now you're holding your newborn baby, a sweet, strong-willed small package of amazing resilience, personality, and love. Sure, there will be some tough moments, but nothing that you, a lesbian who so badly wanted a baby, can't handle. It's been wonderful to stand behind you during your journey to mamahood, and I'm proud to have been part of your process. I wish you all the joy and happiness in the world. After coming this far, you certainly deserve it! Remember, motherhood is not a final destination, but a journey—for you, your partner if you have one, and your baby. Enjoy the ride.

Chapter

13

Resources

Lesbian-Friendly Sperm Banks and Clinics

The development of the Internet has made it easy for most women to quickly get detailed information about fertility issues and sperm banks. This is a huge advantage, both in how fast you can now access information and in how detailed it can be. If you do not have Internet access at home, check your local library to see if they provide computers with free online access. Many cities have Internet cafes that allow you to pay by the minute for online access. If you have no access to any computer, or simply do not want to use one, see below for the addresses and phone numbers of most lesbian-friendly sperm banks. Most will still send you information packets by mail and answer brief questions by phone.

While the following list does not include every sperm bank in existence, and is not limited to the ones used by lesbians, these banks are heavily favored by lesbians and single women. Many also do sperm banking if you want to use a friend as a known donor for directed deposits. Most sperm banks offer the services of fertility counselors, and many offer inseminations on site. Most of these banks provide both unknown donors and donors who are willing to be known to the child. Identity-release programs typically require children to be 18 before they can meet their biological donor father.

Sperm Banks

California Cryobank
1019 Gayley Avenue
Los Angeles, CA 90024
(800) 231–3373
www.cryobank.com
Extremely detailed and up-to-date
website, with donor choices updated
every hour!

Fairfax Cryobank
3015 Williams Drive, Suite 110
Fairfax, VA 22031
(800) 338–8407
www.fairfaxcryobank.com

Midwest Sperm Bank
4333 Main Street
Downer's Grove, IL 60515
(603) 810–1201
www.midwestspermbank.com
Informative website, and they offer
free shipping to all Chicago area customers, via courier.

Pacific Reproductive Services
444 De Haro Street, Suite 222
San Francisco, CA 94107
(415) 487–2288
(888) 469–5800
www.hellobaby.com
Run by women. They offer inseminations on site, have "yes" donors
(donors who are willing to be known
to the child), and are lesbian friendly.

Rainbow Flag Health Services and
Sperm Bank
(510) 521–7737
Leland@gayspermbank.com
www.gayspermbank.com
Owned by a gay man and father. This
bank's donors are primarily gay men. It
is the only bank that gives the mother
the identity of the biological father
when the child is three months old, so
your child can meet and develop a
comfortable relationship with his
donor long before the typical donor
release age, 18 years. You can also
meet the other families whose children
are half siblings of your child, and your
child can grow up knowing them as
family members or special friends.
Located in Alameda, California. They
now ship internationally. And yes, this
is the sperm bank that I used. To use
their services, you must agree not to
perform circumcision on male (or
female) children. They post a female-
child birthrate of 56 percent.

ReproMed Limited
56 Aberfoyle Crescent, Suite 209
Etobicoke, Ontario M8X 2W4
Canada
(877) 249–4282
info@repromedltd.com
www.repromedltd.com
Popular Canadian sperm bank.

Sperm Bank of California
2115 Milvia Street
Berkeley, CA 94704
(510) 841–1858
www.thespermbankofca.org
This company pioneered the donor
identity release program, they are one
of the oldest, and they are the only
nonprofit sperm bank in the U.S. Run
by women, many of them dykes.
Highly informative website and knowledgeable, caring staff. The downside:
They only ship to doctors, so if you
want to do a home insemination, you
must be under a doctor's supervision.

Xytex Corporation
1100 Emmett Street
Augusta, GA 30904
(800) 277–3210
xytex@xytex.com
www.xytex.com
After you sign up with them, you can
go to their website to view photos of
their donors both as babies and as
grown men. Many lesbians have told
me they've had a very comfortable
time using this bank.

Health Clinics

Fenway Community Health Center
7 Haviland Street
Boston, MA 02115
(617) 267–0900
www.fenwayhealth.org
They do inseminations, but you must
purchase the sperm separately from an
approved bank and have it shipped to
them directly.

Lyon-Martin Women's Health Services
1748 Market Street, Suite 201
San Francisco, CA 94102
Clinic: (415) 565–7767
www.lyon-martin.org
Community-based health center serving primarily the San Francisco lesbian
community. They provide fertility information and referrals.

Online Resources for Expectant or Current Moms

When you are trying to conceive, the Internet can truly be your friend. It's a perfect tool for seeking support, bonding with others, and tracking down all sorts of information. You can spend hundreds of hours surfing lesbian-friendly and single-mom-friendly websites, chat rooms, LISTSERVs, and blogs. It would be impossible for the following list to be comprehensive, given the amount of information now online; and the volume increases daily. Even a simple Google search for "lesbian motherhood" turns up pages of entries. All I can promise is that the following information will start you on your way—the rest is up to you. Bear in mind that all these sites include links to other sites, so happy surfing!

Advocacy for Lesbian Mothers

Family Pride Coalition
www.familypride.org
The preeminent organization advocating for the rights of families headed by lesbians and gays.

Information for Lesbian Moms

The Lesbian Mom's Webpage
www.lesbian.org/moms/index.htm
Although some pages on this site are out of date, it's still a good reference for women starting this journey. Includes topics such as insemination and what names the children in our families use to call their (two) moms.

Proud Parenting
www.proudparenting.com

Gay Parent magazine
www.gayparentmag.com

Rainbow Families
www.rainbowfamilies.org

2moms2dads
www.2moms2dads.com

Our Family Coalition
www.ourfamily.org

Alternative Family Matters
www.alternativefamilies.org
Includes information about the Conception Connection Registry, which links opposite-sex glbtq folks, previously unknown to each other, who are interested in coparenting.

Legal Issues

National Center for Lesbian Rights
870 Market Street, Suite 370
San Francisco, CA 94102
(415) 392–6257
www.nclrights.org
Up-to-the-minute legal information for the lesbian community. Court cases and applicable legislation pertaining to parenting are often posted on their site. You can call NCLR for information about lesbian-friendly attorneys in your area.

LISTSERVs

Some LISTSERVs require you to sign up or have a password for access. It's not hard to do, so don't be intimidated if you haven't used the Web before for groups such as these. The following mailing lists and sites are full of information for lesbian moms and mommy-hopefuls:

moms@groups.queernet.org
Send email to this address to get signed up for specific queer lists.

majordomo@queernet.org
Write to this address if you are dealing with fertility issues.

Non–Queer Specific Sites That Include Queer Lists

Urban Baby
www.urbanbaby.com

Pregnancy and Parenting
http://parenting.ivillage.com/

Yahoo
www.yahoo.com
Yahoo has lots of bulletin boards for single moms by choice, lesbian mothers, and mothers of multiples.

Queer Sites That Include Some Parenting Info

Gay.com
www.gay.com

Planet Out
www.planetout.com

Other Sites of Interest for Particular Topics in Fertility and Parenting

Lesbian Health Research Center
www.lesbianhealthinfo.org

The Fertility Shop
www.thefertilityshop.com
Oodles of products and ideas for your path to pregnancy.

Clearblue Easy
www.clearplan.com
For basic fertility info and Clearplan Easy products.

Resolve: The National Infertility Association
www.resolve.org
Lots of infertility advice.

Single Mothers by Choice
www.singlemothersbychoice.com
A good starting point for single moms.

Children of Lesbians and Gays Everywhere
www.colage.org
Sponsors events for glbtq families and friends, and provides networking opportunities and support for the children of gay men and lesbians.

FertilityPlus
www.fertilityplus.org
Lots of fertility info, including sites and mailing lists dealing with miscarriage, DES daughters, multiples, and conceiving as an overweight woman (OASIS). Here you can find more information about some controversial topics mentioned in this book, such as taking Robitussin to thin out fertile mucus.

Hip Mama
www.hipmama.com
The holy mother site for funky and teen moms.

Mamaphonic
www.mamaphonic.com
For the young and hip crowd.

Ariel Gore
www.arielgore.com
From the creator of Hip Mama.

Blogs

More and more personal blogs (weblogs) are being published online. Recent estimates put the number of parenting blogs alone at more than 8,000! There are some queer ones in the bunch. "The Other Mother" is one I like. It's written by Robin, nonbiological lesbian mom to Pearl, the cute little girl she and her partner are raising. It's updated frequently and always has great new pictures of Pearl. Robin is trying to keep track of the growing number of lesbian family blogs out there, so use her site as a launching pad to find them. You can surf directly from her site's recommended blog list.

www.theothermother.typepad.com/blog

Insemination Supplies

Check sperm bank and fertility websites for insemination supplies. Drugstore sites such as www.thefertilityshop.com also carry supplies. Dry ice must be purchased locally, as it usually lasts no more than a day.

Awakenings Birth Services
P.O. Box 14282
San Francisco, CA 94114
www.awakeningsbirthservices.com
You can order plastic speculums from Awakenings Birth Services. The cost is $12 per speculum, including shipping to a U.S. address ($14 in U.S. currency for shipping to Canadian addresses). Make checks payable to Deborah Simone. No phone calls or credit card orders.

Midwives, Doulas, and Birth Centers

How do you find a lesbian or lesbian-friendly midwife or doula? Start by contacting these organizations.

Doulas of North America (DONA)
(888) 788–DONA
www.dona.org

Midwives Alliance of North America (MANA)
www.mana.org

North American Registry of Midwives
(888) 842–4784
www.narm.org

DoulaWorld.com
www.Doulaworld.com

National Association of Childbearing Centers
www.Birthcenters.org
A state-by-state listing of birth centers, not necessarily all lesbian friendly.

Again, remember that these online listings are only the beginning of what you will find with just a bit of effort. The more you seek and surf, the more you shall find.

Books

My Top Picks

If you'll have only a few other pregnancy and parenting books besides this
one on your shelf, these are the others
I'd recommend:

1. *Considering Parenthood*
   by Cheri Pies
   Spinsters Ink

This is the quintessential workbook for
deciding whether you are ready to be
a lesbian parent. I owned it long
before I starting trying to get pregnant.
The downside here is that you can get
so caught up in processing every
aspect of being the perfect parent at
the perfect time that you might wait
too long to just go ahead and do it.
That almost happened to me.

2. *The Queer Parent's Primer*
   by Stephanie Brill
   New Harbinger Press

While most of this book is applicable
after your child is born, the early chapters "Establishing and Celebrating Your
Family" and "The Foundation of
Healthy Parenting" are worth reading
very seriously in your pregnancy's early
stages. In particular, I found her sections on breastfeeding and the biological mother's important connection to
the child a brave stance in this age of
"equal" coparenting (both in lesbian
couples and lesbians sharing coparenting with gay men).

3. *Women in Love: Portraits of Lesbian
   Mothers & Their Families*
   by Barbara Seyda with Diana
   Herrera
   Bulfinch Press

Technically a coffee-table book, this
lovely photo album of lesbian families
includes moving personal statements
by the women and children featured
in the photographs. A personal favorite
of mine.

4. *The Complete Book of Pregnancy
   and Childbirth*
   by Sheila Kitzinger
   Alfred A. Knopf

The most thoughtful of the mainstream
pregnancy books, written by a respected
childbirth educator and midwife. Lots
of photos and medical information as
well as respectful coverage of hospital
and home birth. New terminology
throughout, replacing "husband" and
"father" with "birthing partner."

5. *Your Pregnancy Week by Week*
   by Glade B. Curtis and Judith
   Schuler
   Da Capo Press

Excellent week-by-week information
about your child's development in
utero, and how the baby's development affects and is affected by the
mother's health and well-being. For
detail queens like me, who will savor
every little tidbit of information.

6. *Wanting a Child*
   edited by Jill Bialosky and Helen
   Schulman
   Farrar, Straus and Giroux
Satisfy your itch for a baby by reading
this collection of writing by other
parental hopefuls—including one lesbian couple.

7. *Buying Dad: One Woman's Search
   for the Perfect Sperm Donor*
   by Harlyn Aizley
   Alyson Publications
Written by a partnered lesbian, a first-
person account of how she and her
girlfriend conceived with donor sperm.
One of the first such personal accounts.

8. *The Nursing Mother's Companion*
   by Kathleen Huggins
   Harvard Common Press
Yes, you will need a book on breastfeeding, and this is the one you should
have on hand—before the baby is
born. Extremely empathetic and
detailed. A necessity if you plan to
breastfeed.

9. *The Baby Book*
   by William and Martha Sears
   Little, Brown and Company
Simply the best book on newborn
care. Covers every possible topic of
baby care, from your first days with a
newborn to the advantages of attachment parenting to baby ailments and
how to treat them. This book was my
parenting bible in my daughter's first
year, answering every conceivable
question and coaching me gently in
how to become the best parent I could
be. Ask for this book at your baby
shower.

10. *A Legal Guide for Lesbian & Gay
    Couples*
    by Hayden Curry, Denis Clifford,
    and Frederick Hertz
    Nolo Press
Sections on parenting issues, continually updated both in book format and
in online supplements.

Other Books Worth a Peek During Your Pregnancy

SPECIFICALLY LESBIAN

*The Complete Lesbian & Gay Parenting
Guide*
by Arlene Istar Lev
Berkeley
Enjoyable reading on the issues of
parenting for gay men and lesbians.

*The Essential Guide to Lesbian
Conception, Pregnancy, and Birth*
by Kim Toevs and Stephanie Brill
Alyson Publications
Written by lesbian midwives.

*Home Fronts: Controversies
in Nontraditional Parenting*
edited by Jess Wells
Alyson Publications
Personal pieces on queer parenthood.

Lesbians Raising Sons: An Anthology
edited by Jess Wells
Alyson Publications
This anthology will be comfort reading
for dykes facing the unique challenges
of raising boy children.

*The Room Lit By Roses: A Journal of
Pregnancy and Birth*
by Carole Maso
Counterpoint Press
A lesbian novelist's poetic account of
longing for and having a child.

STRAIGHT BUT WORTHWHILE

Bedrest
by Sara Bilston
HarperCollins
A (straight) novel about surviving
bedrest, written by a mom who did.

Being Born
by Sheila Kitzinger, photos by Lennart
Nilsson
Grosset & Dunlap
An amazing book of stunning in utero
photographs of a developing baby,
from simple cell to birth.

*Birthing from Within: An Extra-Ordinary
Guide to Childbirth Preparation*
by Pam England
Partera Press
Looks at pregnancy as a spiritual, emo-
tional, and physical journey.

The Everything Baby Names Book
by Lisa Shaw
Adams Media
My favorite baby name book, it features all types of names and their
meanings.

*From Conception to Birth:
A Life Unfolds*
by Alexander Tsiaras, with text by
Barry Werth
Doubleday
Want more photos and information on
what life looks like inside the womb?
This incredible coffee-table book of
conception and pregnancy photographs will appeal to the truly
obsessed.

*Helping the Stork: The Choices and
Challenges of Donor Insemination*
by Carol Frost Vercollone, Heidi Moss,
and Robert Moss
Wiley
Straight but empathetic; by lesbian-
friendly authors.

The Hip Mama Survival Guide
by Ariel Gore
Hyperion
Gore's alternative viewpoint is a welcome relief from the starchy, white,
middle-class perspective of most
pregnancy/parenting books. Specific
information for lower-income women.
Check out Ariel's websites: www.hip-
mama.com and www.arielgore.com.

Homebirth
by Sheila Kitzinger
Dorling Kindersley (out of print but
available used, online)

Meditations for New Mothers
by Beth Wilson Saavedra
Workman Publishing
I loved this little meditation book's
gentle reflections on new motherhood.

The Mommy Book
by Todd Parr
Little, Brown and Company
My favorite alternative mommy picture
book, written and illustrated by a gay
man.

The Multiple Pregnancy Sourcebook
by Nancy Bowers
McGraw-Hill

Operating Instructions: A Journal of My Son's First Year
by Anne Lamott
Fawcett Columbine
This journal-like memoir is one of my favorite books.

Parenting Guide to Pregnancy and Childbirth
by Paula Spencer
Ballantine Books
Covers every imaginable aspect of pregnancy, with good photos and illustrations.

Rediscovering Birth
by Sheila Kitzinger
Pocket Books
Lovely look at birth around the world. You'll feel part of a global community of women.

Sexy Mamas: Keeping Your Sex Life Alive While Raising Kids
by Cathy Winks and Anne Semans
Inner Ocean Publishing
Lots of empathetic information for moms and moms-to-be on their changing sexuality.

Single Mothers by Choice
by Jane Mattes
Three Rivers Press
For single women who are considering, or have chosen, solo motherhood.

Supernanny: How to Get the Best From Your Children
by Jo Frost
Hyperion
Sage parenting advice from the star of ABC Television's *Supernanny*.

Twice Blessed: Everything You Need to Know About Having a Second Child
by Joan Leonard
St Martin's Press
Very heterosexual in outlook but also very good. Includes info on preparation of siblings, second pregnancy and birth, and how life differs with two children.

Twins to Quints: The Complete Manual for Parents of Multiple Birth Children
by the National Organization of Mothers of Twins, Rebecca Moskwinski, editor
Harpeth House Publishing

Appendix

Basal Body Temperature Chart

Days of Cycle	1	2	3	4	5	6	7	8	9	10	11	12	13	14	15	16	17	18	19	20	21	22	23	24	25	26	27	28	29	30	31	32	33	34	35	36	37	38	39	40	41	42
Date of Month																																										
Spin																																										
Surge																																										
Menstruation																																										

99.0°
.8
.6
.4
.2
98.0°
.8
.6
.4
.2
97.0°

Basal Body Temperature Chart from *The Ultimate Guide to Pregnancy for Lesbians* by Rachel Pepper

Index

receiving blanket, 155, 193, 195
relationships, 7, 10, 15–17, 20–22,
     134–35, 136–38, 165–66, 171,
     244–46; breakups, 87, 165–66,
     245; stress on, 134–35
reproductive endocrinologist, 23, 97,
     98, 99, 106, 119
RESOLVE, 100
Rh antibodies, 143
Rh type, 119
rhinitis of pregnancy, 149–50
"ring of fire," 208, 215–16
Riordan, Maura, 64
Robitussin, 254
Room Lit by Roses, The, 84, 257
roommates, 15–16
rough sex, 175, 176
rubella, 24, 74, 109, 119
runny nose, 149–50

S
safer sex, 22, 54–55
sauna, 133
savings, 14–15
second children, 27, 69, 103, 209,
     259
second-parent adoption, 116, 136–37,
     162–63, 197
second trimester, 141–66, 169
selective reduction, 104–05
self-care, 3, 8, 87
self-esteem, 167–78
Semans, Anne, 5, 38, 170, 171, 172,
     175, 178, 259
semen, 48–49, 51, 54, 73, 74, 75, 76,
     78, 79, 81, 83, 177
sex, during pregnancy, 167–78;
     inducing labor, 174, 177;
     positions, 167, 170, 172, 174,
     175; risk of harming fetus,
     174–77; with men, 84–85
sex drive, 91, 142, 167–71
sex selection, 33–34
sex toys, 174–75
Shaw, Lisa, 190, 258
Shields, Brooke, 230, 231
shortness of breath, 151–52, 180
siblings, 69, 104, 163–64, 250, 259

sickle-cell anemia, 24, 74, 144
Sidelines, 186
SIDS (sudden infant death syndrome),
     243
Simone, Deborah, 5, 173, 218, 254
Slater, Lauren, 132
sleep, 127, 142, 148–49, 198;
     deprivation, 7, 125, 198, 221,
     221, 230, 241–42; positions,
     148–49, 170, 198
sleepers, 155
smell, 37, 73, 112, 123, 126, 176, 243
smoking, 38–39, 115, 133
sonogram, 119–21, 144, 145, 187
special-needs children, 18, 110, 187
speculums, 45, 76, 78, 81, 254
sperm, 47–85; collecting, 51; costs,
     73–78; count, 48, 53, 54, 68, 98;
     fresh, 31, 33, 50, 51, 71, 79, 84;
     frozen, 31, 33, 49, 50, 62,
     74–75, 79, 83; life span, 31, 33;
     mobility, 60; motility, 48, 54, 68,
     79; sorting, 34; shipping, 2–3,
     60–62, 73, 74, 76; spun, 49, 75;
     washed, 49
Sperm Bank of California, 5, 61, 63,
     64, 69, 251
sperm banks, 2–5, 24, 48–50, 54, 56,
     60–71, 73–79, 144, 219,
     249–51; and health screening,
     54, 60–62; and homophobia,
     64–65; laws concerning, 60–62;
     and single women, 2, 60–64, 71
spin, *see* mucus
spina bifida, 129, 144, 145
spinnbarkeit, see mucus, spinny
Spock, Dr., 10
spotting, 36, 46, 112, 178, 185
STIs, 22, 84, 176; *see also* chlamydia,
     gonorrhea, hepatitis, herpes,
     syphilis
Stevens, Franco, 4
stress, 39, 86–87, 92, 97, 134–35,
     165, 188, 219; and conception,
     35, 39, 40, 43, 70, 77, 86–87,
     92, 97; in pregnancy, 134–35,
     165; in parenting, 225–32,
     239–40

About the Author

RACHEL PEPPER is an award winning journalist and the book editor at *Curve* magazine. She lives with her daughter Frances in the greater New York area, and works for Yale University.